新工科英语系列教程

Academic English for Medicine

医学学科英语

主　编　刘佳佳　郭书法

副主编　陈典珂　汪田田　马晓婧　王淑娟

编　者　曹　静　陈晓倩　唐　红　刘春芳

卞　佳　万　琼　李雪梅　章洪流

周　彦

清華大学出版社

北　京

内 容 简 介

本教材定位为医学院校学科通用学术英语。每个单元包括主题信息检索与展示、三篇相关主题的阅读文章、课文配套综合训练，以及学术英语技巧学习与分项训练。全书选材来自于权威的科普杂志、医学官方网站和医学学术期刊，兼顾了科普性、学术性、人文性、趣味性和前瞻性。本教材另配有练习答案和 PPT 教学课件，读者可登录“清华社英语在线”（www.tsinghuaelt.com）进行下载。

本教材适用于医学类高等院校学生、医务工作者以及医学英语爱好者。

图书在版编目（CIP）数据

医学学科英语 / 刘佳佳，郭书法主编. —北京：清华大学出版社，2023.8
新工科英语系列教程
ISBN 978-7-302-62464-6

Ⅰ. ①医…　Ⅱ. ①刘…　②郭…　Ⅲ. ①医学－英语－高等学校－教材　Ⅳ. ①R

中国国家版本馆 CIP 数据核字（2023）第 013871 号

责任编辑：倪雅莉
封面设计：陈国熙
责任校对：王凤芝
责任印制：丛怀宇

出版发行：清华大学出版社
网　址：http://www.tup.com.cn, http://www.wqbook.com
地　址：北京清华大学学研大厦A座　　**邮　编：**100084
社 总 机：010-83470000　　**邮　购：**010-62786544
投稿与读者服务：010-62776969, c-service@tup.tsinghua.edu.cn
质量反馈：010-62772015, zhiliang@tup.tsinghua.edu.cn
印 装 者：天津安泰印刷有限公司
经　销：全国新华书店
开　本：185mm×260mm　　**印　张：**15.25　　**字　数：**348 千字
版　次：2023 年 8 月第 1 版　　**印　次：**2023 年 8 月第 1 次印刷
定　价：65.00 元

产品编号：089834-01

前言
Preface

随着医学的不断发展，医学学术国际交流日益频繁，需要医学专业技术人员熟练地使用国际通用语言——英语，阅读英文文献、参加国际学术会议、在国际期刊上发表研究成果等，这无疑给广大的医务工作者及医学专业学生带来了很大的挑战。

2018 年，教育部、国家卫生健康委员会和国家中医药管理局在《关于加强医教协同实施卓越医生教育培养计划 2.0 的意见》中提出“要夯实医学生全面发展的宽厚基础，提升医学生临床综合能力，培育医学生临床科研潜质，拓展医学生国际视野，培养少而精、高层次、高水平、国际化的医学未来领军人才”的号召，这就需要医学生积极提升自身的科研素养，不断提高自身的医学英语水平。《大学英语教学指南》（2020 版）中也明确提出各高校应以需求分析为基础，根据学校人才培养目标和学生成长需要，开设体现学校和专业特色的专门用途英语课程，以增强学生使用英语进行学术交流、从事专业工作的能力，提升学生学术和职业素养。因此，具备较高的医学英语水平是医学生成为卓越医生的必要条件。

本教材是为加快培养适应和引领新一轮科技革命和产业变革的卓越新医科医学人才而编写的医学学术英语教材。作为安徽省一流教材建设项目（2021yljc088）成果，本教材依托省级专业英语教学团队（2020jxtd168），旨在全方位培养医学生的医学学术英语能力。除了面向高等医学院校学生，本教材也适用于需要提高医学英语水平的广大医务工作者，以及对医学感兴趣又想提高英语水平的医学英语爱好者等。

本教材围绕立德树人的根本任务，充分融入课程思政理念和内容。除了注重医学英语知识学习和技能提升，本教材还融入 inestimable value of nursing、mental health care for university students 和 cancer care 等思政主题元素，帮助学生树立正确的世界观、人生观和价值观。全书着眼于医学发展，研究医学与人文的关系，关注医学热点（比如 pandemic 和 medical ethics 等），共分为八个单元，单元主题包括 Pandemic、Medicine、Nursing、Mental Health、Food and Nutrient、Drug、Cancer 和 Medical Ethics。每单元主要包含以下内容：

1. 单元主题检索与展示：这部分给出 5 个单元主题词让学生先行检索，并用口头汇报的方式进行课堂展示。

2. 三篇围绕单元主题的阅读文章：这些文章选自权威的科普杂志［比如 *Scientific American*（《科学美国人》）、*The Economics*（《经济学人》）等］、权

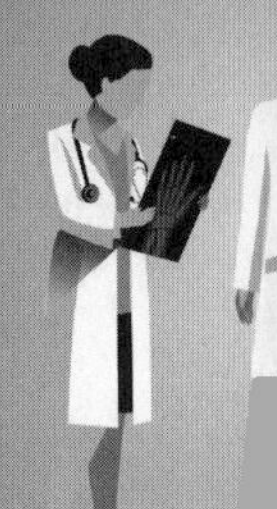

威医学网站（比如世界卫生组织官方网站等），以及权威医学期刊（比如《柳叶刀》《新英格兰医学期刊》等）。全书选材兼顾了科普性、学术性、人文性、趣味性和前瞻性。

3. 课文配套综合训练：围绕单元主题和阅读材料设计了阅读理解、通用及医学专业学术词汇和搭配、翻译等练习。

4. 学术英语技巧学习与分项训练：包含学术英语听力技巧与练习（每单元两篇听力材料，其中一篇选自 TED 演讲）、学术英语阅读技巧与练习，以及学术英语写作技巧与练习。

基于以上内容，本教材重点训练医学生检索、汲取、处理和表达信息的能力；丰富学生通用学术及医学专业学术词汇量；提升学术阅读、学术听说及学术写作能力与技巧。将语言知识的吸收和语言交际能力的培养充分结合起来，以全面培养学习者的医学学术英语技能，进一步增强他们的学术英语交流能力，为其今后更深入的医学专业学习和工作交流做好学术英语能力上的准备。

感谢教材总主编蔡基刚教授在本教材编写过程中悉心、专业的指导，感谢省级教学研究项目（2019jyxm248）、新医科外语课程思政虚拟教研室（2021xnjys019）、新医科课程思政建设示范中心（2021kcszsfzx014）和教育部产学合作协同育人项目（202102430022）项目组成员对教材编写所付出的努力，感谢兄弟院校的同行和清华大学出版社在本教材编写及出版过程中的倾情付出。由于编者水平有限，编写时间仓促，书中如有纰漏，恳请读者见谅并指正。

刘佳佳

2023 年 2 月

目录
Contents

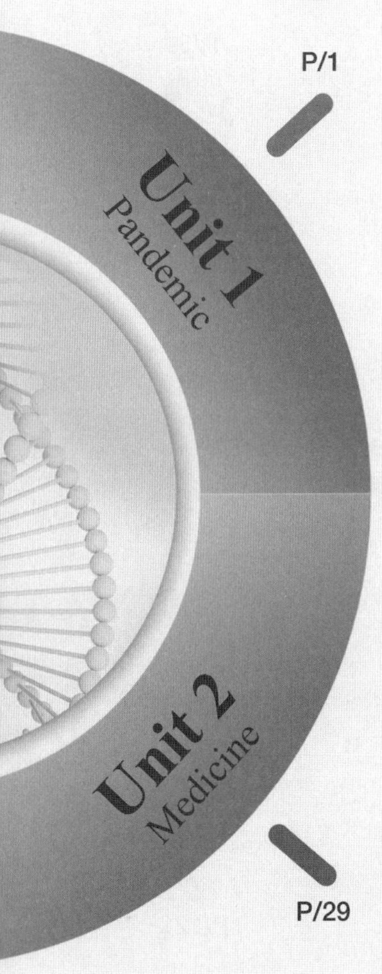

Part A Information Searching and Delivering 2
Part B Text Understanding 2
Passage 1 Pandemics—What Everyone Needs to Know .. 2
Passage 2 A Universal Flu Vaccine Is Vital 5
Passage 3 Wearing Face Masks in the Community During the COVID-19 Pandemic: Altruism and Solidarity 8
Part C Integrated Exercises 11
Part D Academic Skills 18
Academic Listening Skill: Recognizing Main Ideas and Supporting Details 18
Academic Reading Skill: Medical Terminology 23
Academic Writing Skill: Topic Sentence and Supporting Details 25

Part A Information Searching and Delivering 30
Part B Text Understanding 30
Passage 1 Medicine 30
Passage 2 What Are the Benefits and Advantages of Telemedicine? 33
Passage 3 Interpreting the Language of Traditional Medicine 36
Part C Integrated Exercises 40
Part D Academic Skills 47
Academic Listening Skill: Recognizing Signal Words 47
Academic Reading Skill: Skimming and Scanning 52
Academic Writing Skill: How to Write Definitions 55

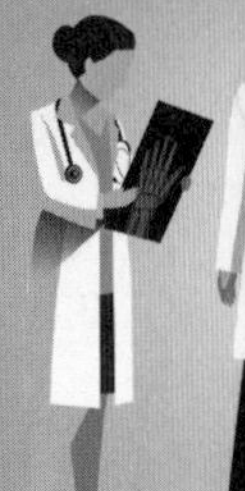

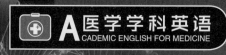

Part A Information Searching and Delivering 60
Part B Text Understanding 60
Passage 1 Men in Nursing: The Challenges in Caregiving... 60
Passage 2 2020: Unleashing the Full Potential of Nursing... 64
Passage 3 If Nurses Nurse, Why Don't Doctors Doctor? ... 66
Part C Integrated Exercises 70
Part D Academic Skills 77
Academic Listening Skill: Finding the Sequence of Events in a Narrative 77
Academic Reading Skill: Signal Words 81
Academic Writing Skill: Comparison and Contrast 83

Part A Information Searching and Delivering 90
Part B Text Understanding 90
Passage 1 Mental Health and Mental Disorders 90
Passage 2 No Physical Health Without Mental Health: Lessons Unlearned? 94
Passage 3 Mental Health Care for University Students: A Way Forward? 96
Part C Integrated Exercises 100
Part D Academic Skills 108
Academic Listening Skill: Making Predictions 108
Academic Reading Skill: Topic Sentences 112
Academic Writing Skill: Problem and Solution 115

Part A Information Searching and Delivering 122
Part B Text Understanding 122
Passage 1 Diet, Nutrition and Inflammatory Bowel Diseases (Excerpt) 122
Passage 2 Fact or Fiction? Feed a Cold, Starve a Fever —The Answer Is Simmering in a Bowl of Chicken Soup 126
Passage 3 Does Lactose Cause Bloating? 128
Part C Integrated Exercises 132
Part D Academic Skills 139
Academic Listening Skill: Making Inferences 139
Academic Reading Skill: Inference Making 142
Academic Writing Skill: Cause and Effect 146

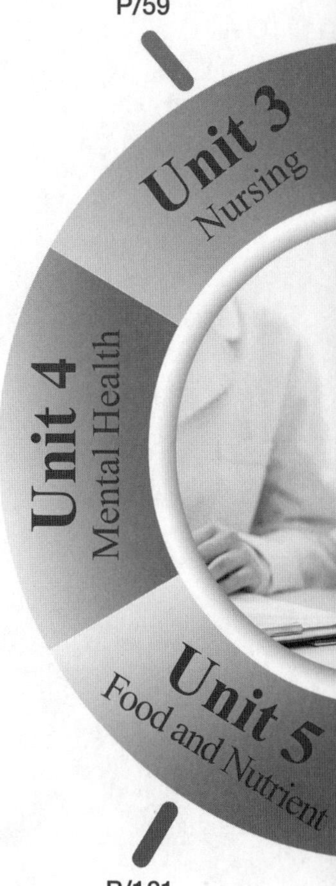

Contents

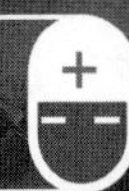

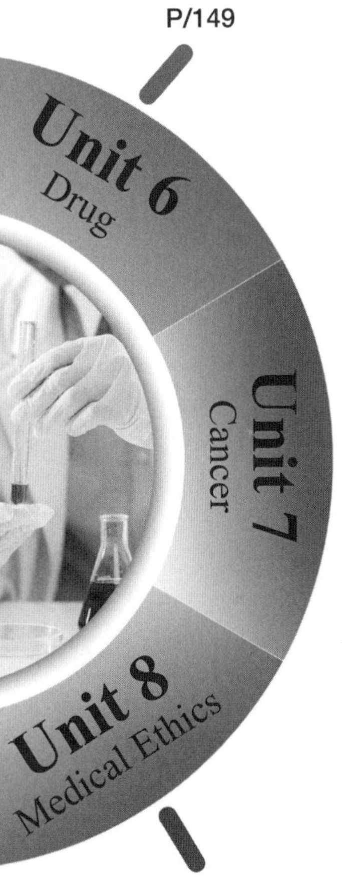

Part A Information Searching and Delivering 150
Part B Text Understanding 150
Passage 1 Medicine's Journey Through the Body 150
Passage 2 When Legal Drugs Harm and Illegal Drugs Help 153
Passage 3 Dealing with Drug Pricing: Not Just One Solution 155
Part C Integrated Exercises 158
Part D Academic Skills 165
Academic Listening Skill: Identifying Numbers 165
Academic Reading Skill: Facts and Opinions 169
Academic Writing Skill: Examples and Statistics 171

Part A Information Searching and Delivering 176
Part B Text Understanding 176
Passage 1 Building a More Resilient Cancer Healthcare System 176
Passage 2 Disability in Cancer Care: Time for Change? 179
Passage 3 Time to Focus on Value-Based Metrics for Cancer Care? 181
Part C Integrated Exercises 185
Part D Academic Skills 193
Academic Listening Skill: Recognizing Cause and Effect Relationship 193
Academic Reading Skill: Arguments and Evidences 198
Academic Writing Skill: Quoting and Paraphrasing 201

Part A Information Searching and Delivering 206
Part B Text Understanding 206
Passage 1 Introduction to Medical Ethics (Excerpt) 206
Passage 2 Palliative Care—A Shifting Paradigm 210
Passage 3 A Genetically Augmented Future 213
Part C Integrated Exercises 216
Part D Academic Skills 223
Academic Listening Skill: Summarizing 223
Academic Reading Skill: Tables and Figures 227
Academic Writing Skill: Summarizing 232

Unit 1

Pandemic

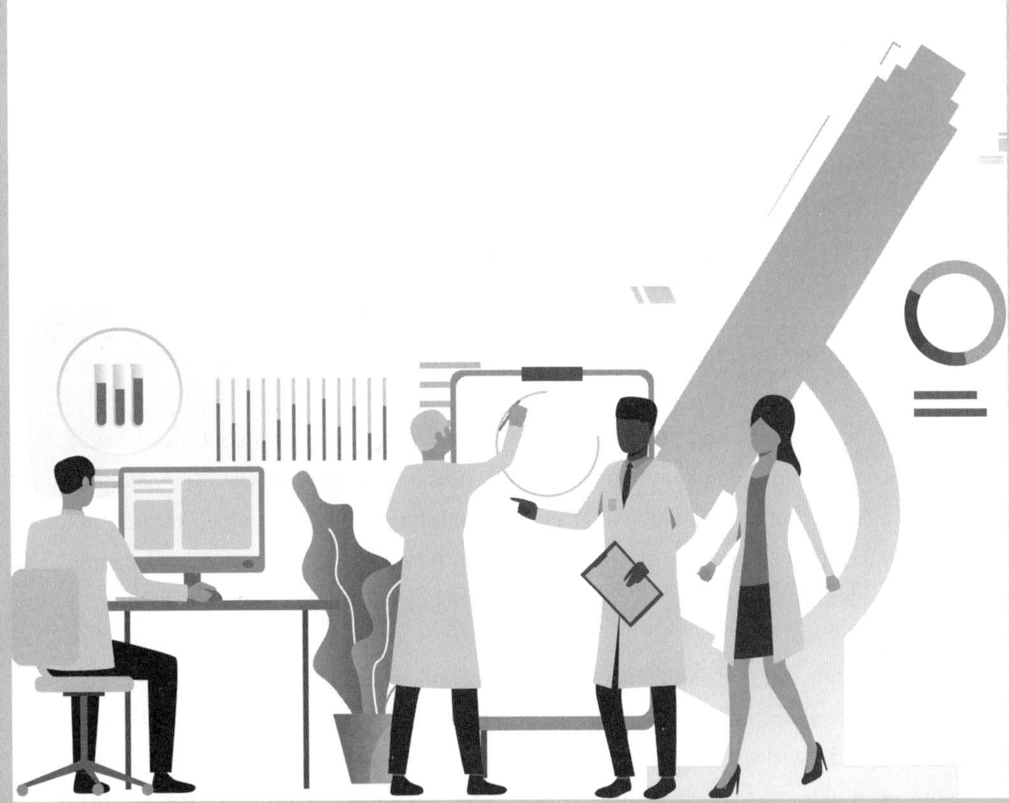

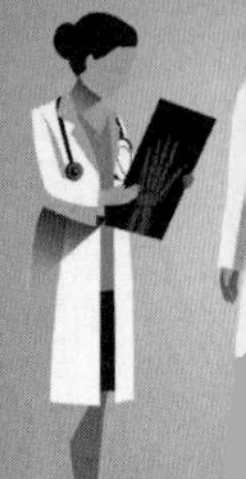

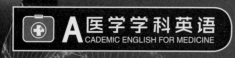

Part A Information Searching and Delivering

I. Surf on the Internet and find information about the following pandemics before class.

1. the Black Death
2. tuberculosis (TB)
3. HIV/AIDS
4. SARS
5. swine flu

II. Make a presentation based on the information you've searched.

Part B Text Understanding

Passage 1 Pandemics—What Everyone Needs to Know

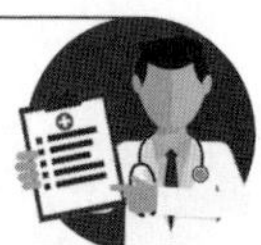

What is the exact definition of pandemic?

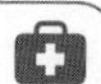

A novel infection—new and previously unconfronted—that spreads globally and results in a high incidence of morbidity (sickness) and mortality (death) has, for the past 300 years or more, been described as a "pandemic". The word derives from the Greek *pan-* (which means "across") and *demos* (which means "people" or "population"). A pandemic spreads across all people. The 1918–1919 flu virus disseminated worldwide, without regard to race, location, cultural belief system, or social status.

There is, though, some disagreement about how and when the term should be used. Until very recently, evidence of contagion monitored by the rapid spread of unfamiliar and generally distressing symptoms was still the main measure of a new, readily transmitted disease. Before the germ theory of infection became established in the mid-to-late nineteenth century and for many

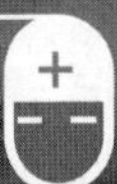

years thereafter, the prevalence and severity of clinical impairment was all that we had to go on. That situation has now vastly changed, with the 150-year-and-continuing—progression in the unraveling of infectious diseases and the incredible advances in both understanding and diagnostic technology that advanced gradually until the 1980s or so, to gather ever increasing momentum with the molecular biology revolution of the past 30 years. Now, modern science provides us with tests that enable the identification of any causative organism both quickly and definitively.

This capacity for rapid diagnosis means that we no longer rely solely, if at all, on seeing severe symptoms. A readily detectable infectious agent that, like the 2009 swine flu virus, tends to cause relatively mild disease in most people but spreads rapidly around the planet will, according to currently used criteria, legitimately be described as causing a pandemic. That's where confusion can arise: the general sense is that "pandemic" is synonymous with catastrophe. With both the media and the broader population ultimately perceiving that the 2009 swine flu pandemic was no more dangerous than the familiar, recurring, "seasonal" influenza epidemics, many had the sense that the regulatory and public health authorities had vastly overstated the level of risk.

Who declares a pandemic?

Pandemic infections are global problems that cannot be dealt with exclusively by individual nation-states. Epidemiologists, statisticians, and other professionals working at the World Health Organization (WHO) based in Geneva, Switzerland, have the responsibility for declaring whether or not a pandemic is occurring. Charged with monitoring and protecting human health everywhere on the planet, the WHO is one of the better functioning agencies of the United Nations. Unlike some UN operations, it rarely attracts the ire of political extremists and xenophobes. Even so, on June 11, 2009, WHO's decision to raise the level of influenza pandemic alert from Phase 5 to Phase 6 ultimately stimulated a great deal of negative media commentary. This first flu pandemic of the twenty-first century just wasn't up to expectations! Nonetheless, working with various national bodies, the WHO generally does a good job, and the 2009 influenza experience illustrates the various stages that culminate in the declaration of a pandemic.

How does the WHO operate?

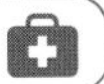

While the central office is in Geneva, the planet is divided for administrative purposes into 6 regions: Africa, Europe, the Eastern Mediterranean, Southeast Asia, the Western Pacific, and the Americas. Each has a WHO office that serves between 11 and 53 different countries, and the division is not strictly geographic. The Regional Office for the Western Pacific, which includes nations as diverse in geography, size, and location as Australia, China, and Tuvalu, is located in Manila, while that for Southeast Asia is in New Delhi. Some Indonesian territories located on a

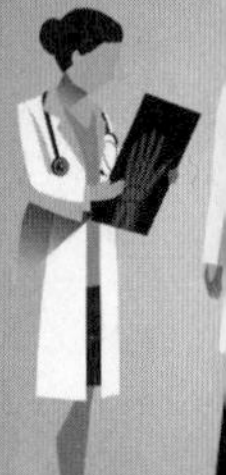

standard global map come under the Southeast Asia office.

With influenza, the WHO defines six grades of Pandemic Alert Phase, based on the incidence of the disease and the extent of spread within and between the various regions. The criteria are published and available on the Web for all to see. A Phase 2 Alert, for example, merely informs public health officials, the media, and anyone who cares to look that a new influenza virus has emerged from some animal reservoir (such as pigs, in the case of the 2009 pandemic) and is causing infection in people. Phase 4 means that human-to-human transmission is at a level where there is a continuing, sustainable outbreak within a community. Phase 5 means that the outbreak has now spread to at least two countries in a particular WHO region. The final Phase 6 Alert is issued when human-to-human spread progresses from one WHO region to a second and significant numbers of people are infected.

This classification system, which depends on the distribution and prevalence of the infection, means that the declaration of a Phase 6 influenza pandemic alert does not basically depend on the virulence, or pathogenicity, of the particular influenza A virus. But, given that the terms "pandemic" and "catastrophe" are synonymous to most people, why not change the definition? The problem is that doing so means coupling two different criteria and deciding ahead of time on outcomes that may not ultimately prove to be valid. For example, an influenza infection that seems to be not too bad when it occurs among those who are adequately housed and fed in a wealthy country may prove to be a true catastrophe for the less fortunate. Differences between rich and poor nations involve more than food and shelter, and include a multitude of factors like the availability of medical oxygen support and rapid access to the appropriate antibiotics for treating secondary bacterial infections that can deliver the coup de grace in a viral pneumonia. Then, apart from any social disadvantage, there is the genetic variation that can distinguish ethnic groups and the threat, particularly with influenza, that the virus may mutate to a more virulent form.

"Pandemic" applies to all populations equally, even when they are not in fact equal. Once a novel pathogen starts to spread rapidly and widely, a pandemic must be declared.

Source: Doherty, P. C. 2013. *Pandemics—What Everyone Needs to Know.* New York: Oxford University Press, pp.42-47.

I. Match the words with their definitions according to Passage 1.

____ 1. epidemic	ⓐ different from anything known before
____ 2. recurring	ⓑ to separate and clarify the elements of sth. mysterious or baffling

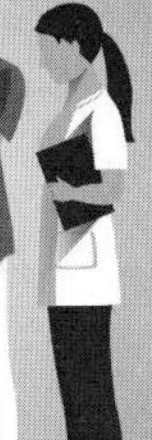

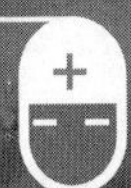

____ 3. impairment	ⓒ the spreading of a disease by people touching each other
____ 4. novel	ⓓ happening more than once, or a number of times
____ 5. culminate	ⓔ (disease) spreading quickly among many people in the same place for a time
____ 6. unravel	ⓕ not severe or acute
____ 7. mutate	ⓖ to end with a particular result, or at a particular point
____ 8. contagion	ⓗ anger
____ 9. ire	ⓘ a condition in which a part of a person's mind or body is damaged or does not work well
____ 10. mild	ⓙ to develop or make sth. develop a new form or structure, because of a genetic change

II. Read Passage 1 and answer the following questions.

1. What's the definition and etymology of pandemic?

   ____

2. What's the general responsibility of the World Health Organization?

   ____

3. Is pandemic synonymous with catastrophe? Why or why not?

   ____

4. What is the basis of the influenza pandemic classification system?

   ____

5. Since the definition of pandemic leads to confusion among people, why hasn't it been changed?

   ____

Passage 2 A Universal Flu Vaccine Is Vital

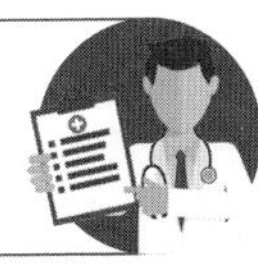

This year the world will mark the 100th anniversary of one of the most devastating infectious disease events in recorded history: the 1918 influenza pandemic, which caused an estimated 50 million to 100 million deaths worldwide.

There were several reasons for the awful toll. First, most people likely had no preexisting immune protection to the brand-new strain that had emerged. Second, this particular virus may have been unusually lethal. Third, crowding and poor sanitation allowed for rampant disease

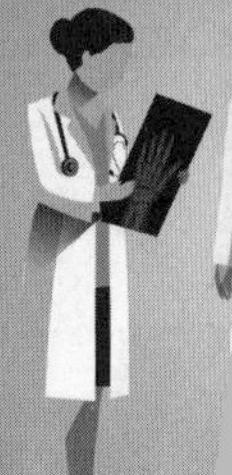

transmission, especially in regions where access to health care was limited. And finally, antiviral drugs and flu vaccines were still decades in the future.

Over the past century we have made substantial advances in all these areas. But we are still unprepared for the inevitable appearance of a virus like the one that struck a century ago. Even an ordinary seasonal flu epidemic will still kill some 12,000 to 56,000 people every year in the US alone. That is because seasonal viruses continually evolve, and although we update our vaccines frequently, they may be only 40 to 60 percent effective. Moreover, seasonal vaccines may provide little or no protection against pandemic flu. Pandemic viruses typically arise from a process referred to as an antigenic shift, in which the new virus acquires, usually from animal influenza viruses, one or more genes that are entirely novel (as seems to have happened in 1918, when all eight pandemic virus genes were novel).

In the years since 1918, three influenza pandemics associated with antigenic shifts occurred: in 1957, 1968 and 2009. In each of these instances, however, the new viruses emerged via the mixing of animal influenza virus genes with those of the 1918-descended viruses already circulating in the human population, which meant that many people were at least partially immune. That, plus lower viral pathogenicity and improvements in public health infrastructure and medical treatment, is what probably led to less catastrophic pandemics.

We must also tackle the issue of "prepandemic" influenza viruses—those that could potentially cause pandemics but that have not (yet) done so. Human infections with avian influenza viruses have occurred with increasing frequency over the past two decades. Prepandemic vaccines against various strains of H5N1 and H7N9 viruses have been developed and in some cases stockpiled; similar to seasonal influenza viruses, however, these avian strains are subject to antigenic drift within their avian hosts. Many of the H7N9 avian viruses that have jumped species from poultry to cause human infections in China in 2016 and 2017 have changed significantly from 2013 avian strains. As a result, the human immune responses elicited by a vaccine developed against the 2013 H7N9 virus may not be effective against 2017 strains.

The remarkable capacity of influenza viruses to undergo antigenic drift or shift to overcome and escape human population immunity leaves us vulnerable to a public health disaster potentially as serious as the 1918 pandemic. To meet this global health challenge, scientists are working to develop "universal influenza vaccines"—new types of inoculations that can provide protection not only against changing seasonal influenza viruses but also against the inevitable pandemic viruses that will emerge in the future.

Recently the National Institute of Allergy and Infectious Diseases convened a workshop with leading experts in the influenza field to address the need for better influenza vaccines. Among many obstacles to developing a universal vaccine, the most formidable is our incomplete understanding of the immune responses that protect people against influenza, including the role of immunity at mucosal surfaces.

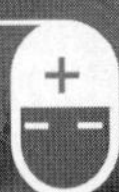

One approach is to design a vaccine to generate antibody responses to parts of the virus that are common to all influenza strains and do not readily change by mutation. It is also crucial to clarify how other parts of the immune system work together with antibodies to protect against influenza. The hurdles in the development of such vaccines are daunting. But we are optimistic that we can apply existing tools and experimental strategies to meet the challenge. As we note the centennial of the 1918 flu pandemic, let us remind ourselves of the importance of this line of research in preventing a repeat of one of the most disastrous events in the history of global health.

Source: Paules, C. I. & Fauci, A. S. 2018. 100 years after the lethal 1918 flu pandemic, we are still vulnerable. *Scientific American, 318*(2): 8.

I. Match the words with their definitions according to Passage 2.

____ 1. antiviral	ⓐ to store a large supply of sth. for future use
____ 2. rampant	ⓑ to appear or come out from somewhere
____ 3. emerge	ⓒ to pass by transmission
____ 4. influenza	ⓓ a group of organisms within a species or variety, characterized by some particular quality
____ 5. centennial	ⓔ of, relating to, or derived from birds
____ 6. strain	ⓕ destroying or inhibiting the growth and reproduction of viruses
____ 7. daunting	ⓖ infectious virus disease causing fever, muscular pain and catarrh
____ 8. descend	ⓗ (of disease, crime, etc.) flourishing excessively
____ 9. avian	ⓘ frightening in a way that makes you feel less confident
____ 10. stockpile	ⓙ the 100th anniversary

II. Read Passage 2 and answer the following questions.

1. What's the historical background of the passage?

____

2. Why are we still unprepared for the appearance of pandemic flu?

____

3. Why might the H7N9 vaccine developed in 2013 be ineffective a few years later?

____

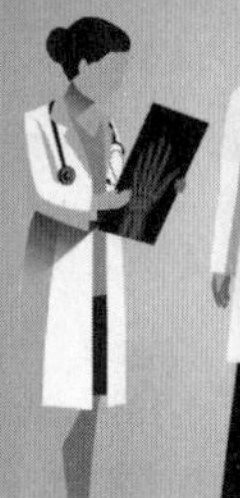

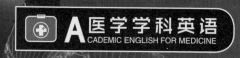

4. According to the author, how to develop "universal influenza vaccines"?

____

5. What is the main idea of the passage?

____

Passage 3 Wearing Face Masks in the Community During the COVID-19 Pandemic: Altruism and Solidarity

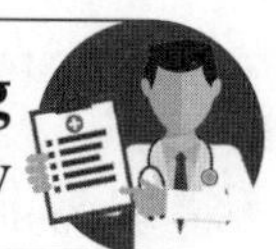

As the coronavirus disease 2019 (COVID-19) pandemic progresses, a debate takes place concerning the use of masks by individuals in the community. We previously highlighted some inconsistency in WHO's initial January, 2020, guidance on this issue. WHO did not recommend mass use of masks for healthy individuals in the community (mass masking) as a way to prevent infection with severe acute respiratory syndrome coronavirus 2 (SARS-COV-2) in its interim guidance of April 6, 2020. Public Health England (PHE) has made a similar recommendation. By contrast, the US Centers for Disease Control and Prevention (CDC) now advises the wearing of cloth masks in public, and many countries require or advise their citizens to wear masks in public places. An evidence review and analysis have supported mass masking in this pandemic. There are suggestions that WHO and PHE are revisiting the question.

People often wear masks to protect themselves, but we suggest a stronger public health rationale be source control to protect others from respiratory droplets. This approach is important because of possible asymptomatic transmissions of SARS-COV-2. Authorities such as WHO and PHE have hitherto not recommended mass masking because they suggest there is no evidence that this approach prevents infection with respiratory viruses including SARS-COV-2. Previous research on the use of masks in non-health-care settings had predominantly focused on the protection of the wearers and was related to influenza or influenza-like illness. These studies were not designed to evaluate mass masking in whole communities. Research has also not been done during a pandemic when mass masking compliance is high enough for its effectiveness to be assessed. But absence of evidence of effectiveness from clinical trials on mass masking should not be equated with evidence of ineffectiveness. There are mechanistic reasons for covering the mouth to reduce respiratory droplet transmission and, indeed, cough etiquette is based on these considerations and not on evidence from clinical trials. Evidence on non-pharmaceutical public health measures including use of masks to mitigate the risk and impact of pandemic influenza was reviewed by a workshop convened by WHO in 2019; the workshop concluded that although there was no evidence from trials of effectiveness in reducing transmission, "there is mechanistic

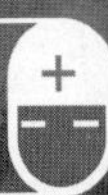

plausibility for the potential effectiveness of this measure", and it recommended that in a severe influenza pandemic use of masks in public should be considered. Dismissing a low-cost intervention (such as mass masking) as ineffective because there is no evidence of effectiveness in clinical trials is potentially harmful.

Another concern is the shortage of mask supply in the community. Medical masks must be reserved for health-care workers. Yet to control the infection source rather than to self-protect, we believe that cloth masks, as recommended by the CDC, are likely to be adequate, especially if everyone wears a mask. Cloth masks can be easily manufactured or made at home and reused after washing. Authorities also worry about correct techniques for wearing, removal, and disposal of face masks, but these techniques could be learned through public education.

Finally, there are concerns that mask wearing could engender a false sense of security in relation to other methods of infection control such as social distancing and handwashing. We are unaware of any empirical evidence that wearing masks would mean other approaches to infection control would be overlooked. It is important, however, to emphasize the importance of this point to the public even if they choose to wear masks.

Mass masking is underpinned by basic public health principles that might not have been adequately appreciated by authorities or the public. First, controlling harms at source (masking) is at least as important as mitigation (handwashing). The population benefits of mass masking can also be conceptualized as a so-called prevention paradox—ie, interventions that bring moderate benefits to individuals but have large population benefits. Seatbelt wearing is one such example. Additionally, use of masks in the community will only bring meaningful reduction of the effective reproduction number if masks are worn by most people—akin to herd immunity after vaccination. Finally, masking can be compared to safe driving: other road users and pedestrians benefit from safe driving and if all drive carefully, the risk of road traffic crashes is reduced.

Social distancing and handwashing are of prime importance in the current lockdown. We suggest mask wearing would complement these measures by controlling the harm at source. Mass masking would be of particular importance for the protection of essential workers who cannot stay at home. As people return to work, mass masking might help to reduce a likely increase in transmission. We encourage consideration of mass masking during the coming phases of the COVID-19 pandemic, which are expected to occur in the absence of an effective COVID-19 vaccine. Finally, this practice could also be useful for control of future influenza epidemics.

Mass masking for source control is a useful and low-cost adjunct to social distancing and hand hygiene during the COVID-19 pandemic. This measure shifts the focus from self-protection to altruism, actively involves every citizen, and is a symbol of social solidarity in the global response to the pandemic.

Source: Cheng, K. K., Lam, T. H. & Leung, C. C. 2020, April 16. Wearing face masks in the community during the COVID-19 pandemic: Altruism and solidarity. *The Lancet*.

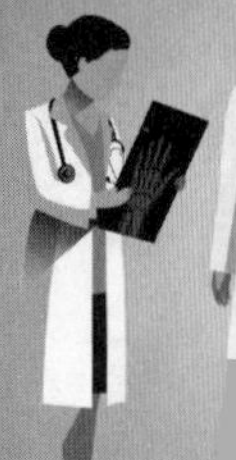

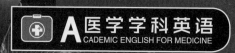

I. Match the words with their definitions according to Passage 3.

____ 1. droplet	ⓐ formal rules of correct and polite behavior in society or among members of a profession
____ 2. lockdown	ⓑ consider sb./sth. not worth thinking or talking about
____ 3. progress	ⓒ a small drop of a liquid
____ 4. etiquette	ⓓ of or at the beginning
____ 5. predominantly	ⓔ (often disapproving) connected with the belief that all things in the universe can be explained as if they were machines
____ 6. dismiss	ⓕ mostly or mainly
____ 7. altruism	ⓖ to go forward in time
____ 8. initial	ⓗ principle of considering the welfare and happiness of others before one's own
____ 9. paradox	ⓘ an emergency protocol to prevent people or information escaping, which usually can only be ordered by someone in command
____ 10. mechanistic	ⓙ a situation or statement which seems impossible or is difficult to understand because it contains two opposite facts or characteristics

II. Read Passage 3 and answer the following questions.

1. What does "mass masking" mean?

____

2. What is the first common concern among people about wearing face masks in the community during the COVID-19 pandemic? How does the author argue that it is unreasonable?

____

3. What is the second common concern among people about wearing face masks in the community during the COVID-19 pandemic? How does the author argue that it is unreasonable?

____

4. What is the third common concern among people about wearing face masks in the community during the COVID-19 pandemic? How does the author argue that it is unreasonable?

____

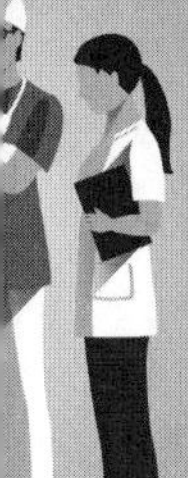

5. What is the main idea of the passage?

___

III. Read the three passages comprehensively and answer the following questions.

1. What is the common theme of the three passages?

___

2. What are the differences among the three passages in terms of topic?

___

3. How does Passage 1 differ from Passage 2 and 3 in terms of the general structure?

___

4. Write a short passage of about 100 words to synthesize the information of the three passages.

___

___

___

___

___

Part C | Integrated Exercises

I. Read the words below, and pay attention to the pronunciation. Use the scale below (1, 2, 3) to give yourself a score for each word. Try to consult your dictionary for the words with score 1.

❶ I don't understand this word.

❷ I understand this word when I see it or hear it, but I don't know how to use it.

❸ I know this word and can use it in my own speaking and writing.

Academic words

□ access	□ adequate	□ assess	□ causative
□ clarify	□ complement	□ convene	□ daunting

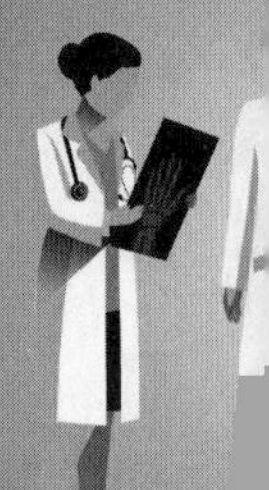

□ descend □ diverse □ elicit □ empirical
□ formidable □ highlight □ hitherto □ hurdle
□ incidence □ mechanistic □ mitigate □ novel
□ outbreak □ overstate □ paradox □ perceive
□ plausibility □ predominantly □ progress □ rampant
□ rationale □ recurring □ regulatory □ solidarity
□ statistician □ stockpile □ tackle □ trial
□ update □ valid □ workshop □ xenophobe

Discipline-specific words

□ acute □ allergy □ antibiotics □ antibody
□ antigenic □ antiviral □ asymptomatic □ bacterial
□ clinical □ contagion □ coronavirus □ epidemic
□ epidemiologist □ flu □ genetic □ germ
□ host □ hygiene □ immune □ impairment
□ infectious □ inoculation □ molecular □ morbidity
□ mortality □ mucosal □ mutate □ organism
□ pathogenicity □ pharmaceutical □ pneumonia □ prepandemic
□ prevalence □ strain □ syndrome □ toll
□ transmission □ vaccine □ virulence □ virus

II. Match each word in the box with the group of words that regularly occur in academic writing.

perceive	elicit	convene	tackle	highlight
stimulate	assess	overstate	clarify	mitigate

1. ______________ pain / environmental effect / poverty
2. ______________ interest / the flow of blood / economic growth
3. ______________ a statement / one's position / the relationship
4. ______________ the case / the risk / the facts
5. ______________ a difficult problem / the inflation / the key issues
6. ______________ the members / the committee /a conference / a special session of congress
7. ______________ an emotional response / a reaction / relevant financial information

8. ______________ the impact / students' ability / a patient's needs
9. ______________ the spelling mistakes / one's skills / the tensions
10. ______________ a change / a tiny figure / the inner nature

III. Study the members of the word families in the table below. Try to work out the meaning in each case according to its prefix or suffix.

The members of a word family	Chinese definitions
diagnose, diagnostic, diagnosis, diagnostically	诊断 (*v.*)、诊断的、诊断 (*n.*)、诊断地
consistent, inconsistent, consistency, inconsistency	
bacterium, bacteria, bacterial, bacteriology	
sustain, sustained, sustainable, unsustainable	
infect, infectious, infection, infector	
circulate, circulatory, circulation	
immune, immunity, immunology, immunize, immunization	
substance, substantial, substantially, substantiality	
pandemic, pandemia, pandemicity	
identify, identifiable, identifier, identification	
vaccine, vaccinal, vaccinate, vaccination, vaccinator	
exclude, exclusive, exclusively, exclusion	
respire, respiratory, respiration, respirator	
adequate, inadequate, adequately, adequacy, inadequacy	
pharmacy, pharmaceutic, pharmaceutical, pharmaceutically	
allergy, allergic, allergen, allergist	
effect, effective, effectiveness, ineffectiveness	
intervene, intervention, interventionist, interventionism	
symptom, symptomatic, asymptomatic, symptomless	
gene, genetic, genetics, geneticist	

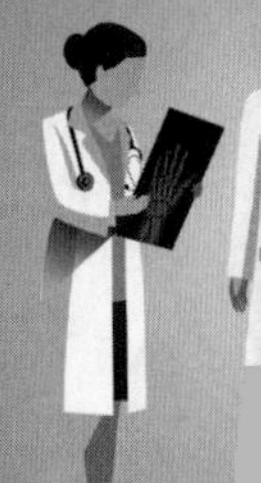

IV. Complete each sentence below with a word from the table above.

1. Smoking places you at serious risk of cardiovascular and ________ disease. (respire)
2. The growing insight into how the immune system distinguishes between internal and external danger is likely to have a ________ impact on therapeutic approaches. (substance)
3. Treatment and prevention of the occurrence of ________ asthma is of great significance. (allergy)
4. The results showed that the ________ breastfeeding rates (EBF) of children under 4 months were 53.7% in the urban area. (exclude)
5. ________ development of environment is closely related to human health. (sustain)
6. One explanation for the ________ of the annual exam in reducing the death rate is that it does little to avert death or disability from acute problems. (effect)
7. In China, it's the focus of the society that how to set up a reasonable, perfect and highly recognized medical malpractice ________ (MMI) system. (identify)
8. Students majoring in ________ investigate disease, its causes and development, and the body's reaction to it. (immune)
9. Poor sanitation leads to ________ diseases that kill more than one and a half million people a year, mostly young children. (infect)
10. Electrocardiograph is an important ________ tool to the heart disease. (diagnose)

V. Choose the word in each list that is not a synonym for the underlined word.

1. <u>disseminate</u>
   A. transmit B. spread C. circulate D. suppress
2. <u>lethal</u>
   A. fatal B. deadly C. nutritious D. mortal
3. <u>compliance</u>
   A. obedience B. abidance C. defiance D. conformity
4. <u>interim</u>
   A. perpetual B. temporary C. transient D. provisional
5. <u>momentum</u>
   A. thrust B. inertia C. impetus D. force
6. <u>engender</u>
   A. breed B. generate C. halt D. cause
7. <u>prime</u>
   A. fundamental B. primary C. chief D. secondary

8. detectable
   A. invisible B. noticeable C. discernible D. observable
9. overlook
   A. neglect B. scrutinize C. disregard D. ignore
10. catastrophe
   A. calamity B. misfortune C. disaster D. blessing

VI. Read the following expressions and sentence patterns aloud and analyze the formality of the structures used.

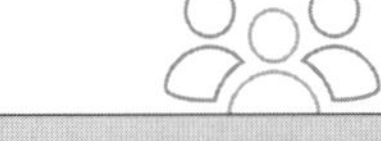

Target sentence patterns

1. A novel infection—new and previously unconfronted—that spreads globally and **results in** a high incidence of morbidity (sickness) and mortality (death) has, for the past 300 years or more, been described as a "pandemic".
2. **There is**, though, **some disagreement about** how and when the term should be used.
3. The 1918–1919 flu virus disseminated worldwide, **without regard to** race, location, cultural belief system, or social status.
4. The prevalence and severity of clinical impairment **was all that** we had to go on.
5. **With** both the media and the broader population ultimately **perceiving that** the 2009 swine flu pandemic was no more dangerous than the familiar, recurring, "seasonal" influenza epidemics, many had **the sense that** the regulatory and public health authorities had vastly overstated the level of risk.
6. The word **derives from** *pan* (which means "across") and *demos* (which means "people" or "population").
7. Pandemic infections are global problems that cannot be **dealt with** exclusively by individual nation-states.
8. "Pandemic" **applies to** all populations equally, even when they are not in fact equal.
9. But **we are** still **unprepared for** the inevitable appearance of a virus like the one that struck a century ago.
10. Differences between rich and poor nations involve more than food and shelter, and include **a multitude of** factors like **the availability of** medical oxygen support and rapid **access to** the appropriate antibiotics for treating secondary bacterial **infections that** can **deliver the coup de**

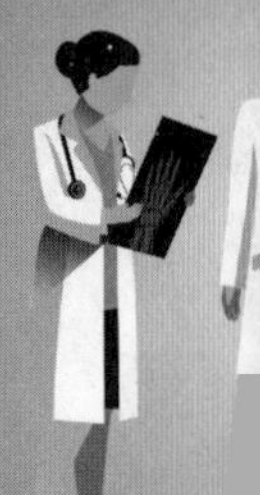

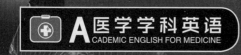

grace in a viral pneumonia.

11. Mass masking **is underpinned by** basic public health **principles that** might not have **been adequately appreciated** by authorities or the public.
12. These avian strains **are subject to** antigenic drift within their avian hosts.
13. New types of **inoculations that** can provide protection **not only** against changing seasonal influenza viruses **but also** against the inevitable pandemic viruses that will emerge in the future.
14. Pandemic viruses typically **arise from** a process **referred to as** an antigenic shift, **in which** the new virus acquires, usually from animal influenza viruses, one or more **genes that** are entirely novel (as seems to have happened in 1918, **when** all eight pandemic virus genes were novel).
15. Social distancing and handwashing **are of prime importance** in the current lockdown.
16. This measure **shifts** the focus **from** self-protection **to** altruism, actively involves every citizen, and is a symbol of social solidarity in the global response to the pandemic.
17. **Yet** to control the infection source **rather than** to self-protect, we believe that cloth masks, **as recommended by** the CDC, **are likely to** be adequate, especially if everyone wears a mask.
18. **Among** many obstacles to developing a universal vaccine, **the most** formidable is our incomplete understanding of the immune responses that **protect** people **against** influenza, **including** the role of immunity at mucosal surfaces.
19. **It is also crucial to** clarify how other parts of the immune system work **together with** antibodies to protect against influenza.
20. We encourage consideration of mass masking during the coming phases of the COVID-19 pandemic, **which** are expected to occur **in the absence of** an effective COVID-19 vaccine.
21. **As** we note the centennial of the 1918 flu pandemic, let us **remind ourselves of** the importance of this line of research in preventing a repeat of one of the most disastrous events in the history of global health.
22. The remarkable capacity of influenza viruses to undergo antigenic drift or shift to overcome and escape human population immunity **leaves us vulnerable to** a public health disaster potentially **as serious as** the 1918 pandemic.
23. **Additionally,** use of masks in the community will only bring meaningful reduction of the effective reproduction number **if** masks are worn by most people—**akin to** herd immunity after vaccination.
24. **Dismissing** a low-cost intervention such as mass masking **as** ineffective because there is no evidence of effectiveness in clinical trials is in our view potentially harmful.
25. **Finally**, there are concerns that mask wearing could **engender a false sense** of security **in relation to** other methods of infection control such as social distancing and handwashing.

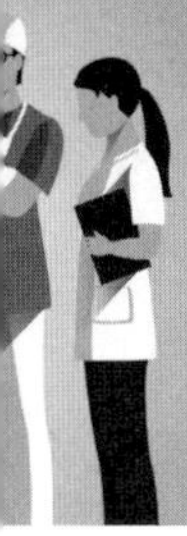

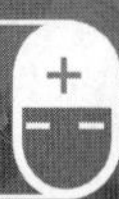

VII. For each of the sentences below, write a new sentence as similar as possible in meaning to the original one, but as formal as possible in style.

1. The mysterious sickness leaves a lot of people dead.

2. It would be a blessing if these 28,000 members of our community got the precious good of health care.

3. Now, modern science makes a simple test to diagnose hyperglycemia possible.

4. Not having enough funds is preventing the UN from monitoring relief.

5. Medical protective suits must be saved for health-care workers.

6. What medical universities or colleges need bear in mind is that passing examinations doesn't mean being educated.

7. Most joints in the body can move freely.

8. Health care workers were not ready to face the magnitude of climate change.

9. Do the findings and therapy of cardiovascular disease have the same influence on men and women?

10. Viability was considered to the same with infectivity.

VIII. Translate the following sentences by using the following words and phrases. Make sure that your English sentences are different from the Chinese versions in terms of structures or orders, but as formal as possible. Then compare yours with your partner's according to the criteria: Whose version is more different and more formal?

1. 医务人员不顾个人安危持续工作。(without regard to)

____

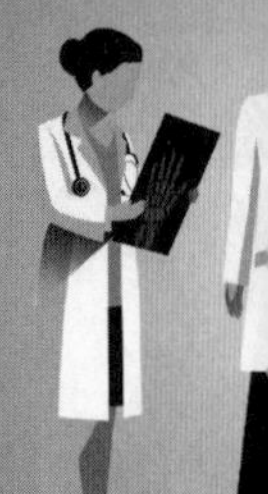

2. 许多医学词汇源自拉丁文。(derive from)

3. 新技术的应用为当今时代医学的飞速发展打下了基础。(be underpinned by)

4. 吸烟者比非吸烟者更容易受到心脏病的侵害。(be subject to)

5. 情绪或精神问题可能是由于身体原因引起的。(arise from)

6. 在休息和恢复阶段，食物摄入至关重要。(be of prime importance)

7. 该政府希望将媒体的注意力从流行病转移到外交政策问题上。(shift from… to…)

8. 病毒侵袭可能会让病人更易受到继发感染。(leave… vulnerable to)

9. 许多人认为色盲是一种很细小的缺陷。(dismiss… as)

10. 一种类似于抑郁的感觉使他不知所措。(akin to)

Part D | Academic Skills

Academic Listening Skill

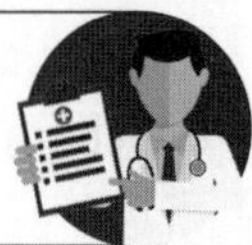

Recognizing Main Ideas and Supporting Details

In academic listening materials, there are main ideas and supporting details. The main idea or main point is the most important or central thought of a paragraph, a section or a whole text. Supporting details provide specific details to support and develop the main point, which contain explanations, examples, reasons and so on. Recognizing main ideas and supporting details is an important skill while listening to an academic material. Note-taking can help you grasp them.

As one of the key note-taking techniques in academic listening, outlining can be used by

listeners to illustrate the relationships between ideas and differentiate main ideas from supporting details, so that you can comprehend listening materials more effectively. There are some methods we can use while outlining, such as using words and phrases instead of the whole sentences. You can organize your notes with headings, subheadings, number lists, symbols, and abbreviations. They can help you to recognize which ideas are main ideas and which are supporting details.

Listening 1

Word bank 

1. coronavirus	1) any of a family (Coronaviridae 冠状病毒科) of large single-stranded RNA viruses that have a lipid envelope studded with club-shaped spike proteins, infect birds and many mammals including humans, and include the causative agents of MERS, SARS, and COVID-19 2) an illness caused by a coronavirus
2. CDC	Centers for Disease Control and Prevention
3. reveal	to make (something secret or hidden) publicly or generally known
4. criteria	a standard on which a judgment or decision may be based
5. executive	one that exercises administrative or managerial control
6. resistance	dislike of or opposition to a plan, an idea
7. cite	to name in a citation
8. terminology	the set of technical words or expressions used in a particular subject
9. syndrome	a group of signs and symptoms that occur together and characterize a particular abnormality or condition

I. Listen to the passage and fill in the blanks. Pay attention to the main ideas and supporting details.

Title
____________ Versus ____________

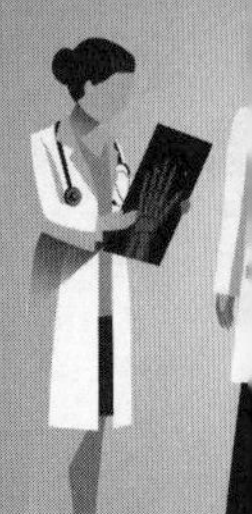

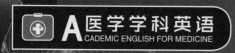

Point 1: What's the difference between them?	
(1) Generally speaking, ______. It's more ______. A pandemic spreads ______ and ______ more people.	
(2) Definition	
According to the CDC, an ______ is an ______, often ______, in the number of ______ of a disease above what is ______ in that ______ in that area.	A ______ is an ______ that has spread over several ______ or ______, usually ______ a large number of people.

Point 2: The reasons why WHO and CDC are sticking with ______ for now	
People	Mike Ryan
Position	the ______ of the WHO world emergencies program
He said	If this were ______, they would have already called it a ______.
	But he further explained their ______ to using the word by ______ concerns that doing so could cause more ______ than ______.
	"For me, I'm not worried about the word. I'm worried about the world's ______ to the word. Will we use it as a call to action? Will we use it to fight? Will we use it to give up?"

Point 3: The related ______ can be ______.
The "demic" part ______ which means ______. "Epi-" in epidemic means ______ or ______. So an "epidemic" is ______. And "pan-" means ______. So a "pandemic" is ______.

II. Listen to the passage again and choose the best answer to each of the following questions.

1 What is the speaker's attitude toward COVID-19?

A Subjective.

B Sympathetic.

C Negative.

D Objective.

❷ **What can you infer from the remarks of Mike?**

A The novel coronavirus has not reached the criteria of pandemic.

B Compared with influenza, the novel coronavirus is merely an epidemic.

C What matters is people's attitude of the novel coronavirus but not the words chosen to define the disease.

D Coronavirus has not been defined as a pandemic because scientists have not known much of it.

Listening 2

Word bank

1. malaria	a serious disease carried by mosquitoes, which causes periods of fever
2. hepatitis	a disease or condition (such as hepatitis A or hepatitis B) marked by inflammation of the liver
3. infect	to make a disease or an illness spread to a person, an animal or a plant
4. genome	the genetic material of an organism
5. co-opt	to take into a group (such as a faction, movement, or culture)
6. replicate	(of a virus or a molecule) to produce exact copies of itself
7. antiretroviral	acting, used, or effective against retroviruses
8. ample	generous or more than adequate in size, scope, or capacity
9. harboring	a place of security and comfort
10. flush	to expose or chase from a place of concealment

**Listen to the passage and take notes while listening.
Then complete the following exercises.**

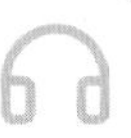

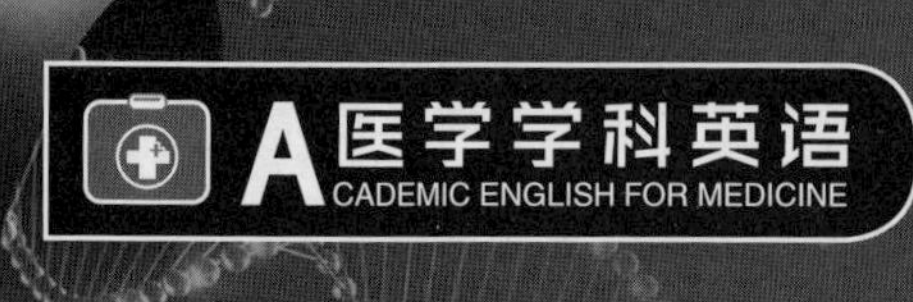

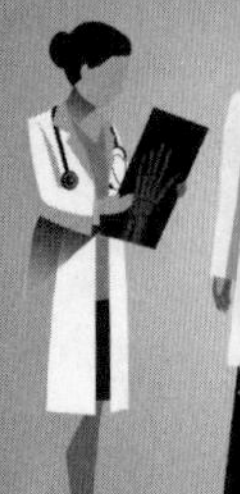

I. Listen to the passage and choose the best answer to each of the following questions.

1 What does the passage mainly talk about?

A How a man was cured of HIV.
B How the drugs for AIDS work.
C The differences between HIV and AIDS.
D The reasons why it's so hard to cure HIV/AIDS.

2 What types of cells does HIV target in human body?

A All types of cells.
B Neurons in the central nervous system.
C T cells that fight against bacterial infections.
D Red blood cells that carry oxygen throughout the body.

3 How long does it typically take when HIV progresses to AIDS without treatment?

A Days.
B Weeks.
C Years.
D Decades.

4 Where does HIV "hide" when it cannot be targeted by antiretroviral therapies?

A In bone marrow stem cells.
B In long-lived neurons in the brain.
C In the DNA of healthy cells.
D None of the above.

5 What is the speaker's attitude about curing AIDS?

A Subjective.
B Sympathetic.
C Negative.
D Positive.

II. Listen to the passage again and fill in the blanks.

1. What will happen at the first stage of HIV infection?

The virus replicates within helper T cells, ________________. During this stage, patients often experience flu-like symptoms, ________________.

2. Why does not everyone in the world have access to the therapies that could save their lives?
   A mix of ________________ makes effective prevention and treatment difficult.

III. Listen to the passage again and decide whether the following statements are true (T) or false (F).

1. Females are not easy to be infected by HIV. ( )
2. HIV can destroy people's immune system. ( )
3. Once every HIV virus is swept from an HIV-positive person's body, he/she can be cured. ( )
4. Sub-Saharan Africa is one of the world's most severely HIV-infected regions. ( )
5. It's possible that AIDS will be cured one day. ( )

Academic Reading Skill

Medical Terminology

Studying medical terminology is as difficult as learning a new language, because they seem strange and complex. Take *ophthalmology* as an example. It means "study of eyes". So, it is important to acquire the word analysis ability. There are mainly five elements worth mentioning: root, suffix, prefix, combining vowel and combining form.

The root is the main part of a word, which endows the term with its essential meaning. For example, the root of the word *ophthalmology* is *ophthalm,* which means "eye". The suffix is the word ending, which either changes the grammatical function of the original word or indicates test, procedure, disorder, etc. The suffix *-logy* means "process of study". The prefix is a small part attached to the beginning of a term, which is often added to change word meanings, like indicating quality, direction, quantity, etc. For example, in the word *hypertension*, *hyper-* means "above", so the whole word means "abnormally high blood pressure". The letter "*o*" often serves as the combining vowel which is added between the root and the suffix or between the root and another root. It should be noted that the combining vowel is removed once the suffix begins with a vowel.

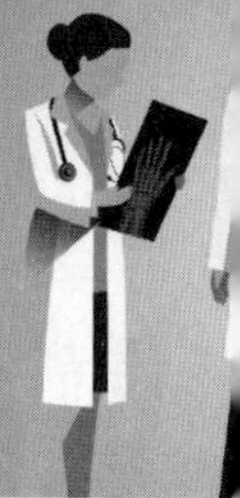

For example, *gastritis* has the suffix *-itis*, which begins with a vowel, so "*o*" is dropped. But it isn't the case when a root begins with vowel. For example, *gastroenterology*, though *enter-* begins with a vowel, there is a combining "*o*" between *gastr-* and *enter-*. Moreover, the combination of root and combining vowel makes a combining form, such as *gastr/o-*.

To analyze a medical term, the rule is to analyze it from the suffix and then go back to the beginning of the term. For example, *epigastric* should be analyzed from *-ic*, which means "pertaining to", and then interpreted from the beginning *epi-* (above) to *gastr-* (stomach), hence pertaining to "above the stomach". In summary, there are 5 important elements in total in medical terms. It is important for students to acquire the skill of identifying and analyzing the medical terms.

I. Analyze the component parts of the terms below and fill in the blanks.

Terminology	Prefix	Root	Suffix
antigen			
arthritis			
mucosal			
antiviral			
tomography			
pathogenicity			
pandemic			

II. Select from the prefixes below to match the numbered words. Write the correct form in the blanks provided.

pneum/o-	pharmac/o-	ophthalm/o-	path/o-	gastr/o-
psych/o-	enter/o-	ren/o-	oste/o-	rhin/o-

1. kidney ________________ 4. bowel ________________
2. mind ________________ 5. medicine ________________
3. bone ________________ 6. lung ________________
7. disease ________________ 9. nose ________________
8. eye ________________ 10. stomach ________________

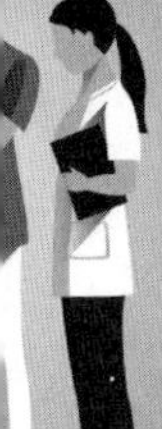

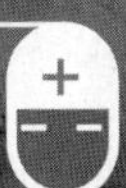

➢ To find more information about medical terminology, you may refer to the following sources.
Chabner, D.-E. 2017. 医学英语教程. 北京：北京大学医学出版社.
孙庆祥. 2020. 医学英语术语实用教程. 上海：复旦大学出版社.

Academic Writing Skill

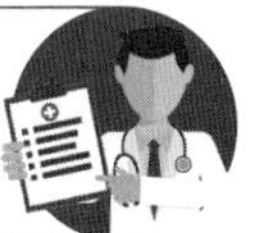

Topic Sentence and Supporting Details

To write a good paragraph, you have to provide your topic sentence with supporting details. Each topic sentence has two elements: a topic and a controlling idea. The controlling idea conveys the author's opinions and feelings about a particular topic. In order to make your topic sentence successful and captivating, you have to make it thorough, concise and brief. However, the supporting details are the information that explains, defines or proves the topic sentence. Supporting details could be: facts (statistics or graphs), statements (quotations or opinions from authorities or experts), examples (comparisons, contrasts, graphs, case studies, illustrations, or predictions), and explanations (clarifications, definitions, sequence of events, causes and effects, or summaries).

In a thesis, it usually consists of several paragraphs with their corresponding topic sentences and supporting details. In order to make the thesis logically organized, transition words are used between paragraphs, topic sentences and supporting details, even between details. For example:

Function	Words and phrases
To add to an idea	and; furthermore; besides; in addition; again; equally important; last but not the least
To compare points	however; in contrast; although; nevertheless; meanwhile; by comparison; on the contrary
To illustrate cause and reason	because; for the reason that; due to; being that; for
To show exception	nevertheless; however; in spite of; yet
To give an example	for example; for instance; to illustrate; in this situation; on this occasion
To show sequence	first; second; third; fourth; then; next

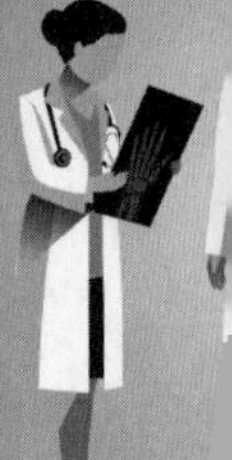

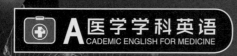

I. Complete the outline of the composition titled "Prevention of Flu".

Prevention of Flu

1 **Topic sentence 1:** A yearly flu vaccine is the best way to protect yourself from flu and its potentially serious complications.
Supporting detail 1: reduce the risk of flu illness by 40%–60%.
Supporting detail 2: ____________________
...

2 **Topic sentence 2:** ____________________
Supporting detail 1: ____________________
Supporting detail 2: ____________________
...

3 **Topic sentence 3:** ____________________
Supporting detail 1: ____________________
Supporting detail 2: ____________________
...

II. Write a composition according to the mind map above. Try to use transition words to make your composition logically organized. (The introductory part and concluding part have been provided here.)

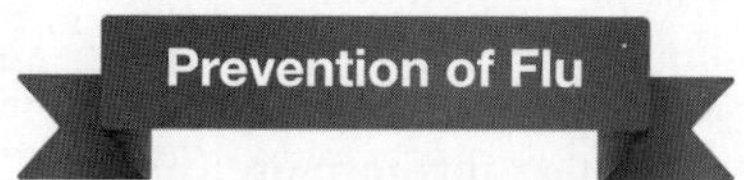

The flu is a respiratory infection that affects many people each year. Anyone can get the virus, which can cause mild to severe symptoms, including fever, body aches, runny nose, coughing, and sore throat. So, it is important for us to know how to prevent the disease.

Firstly, a yearly flu vaccine is the best way to protect yourself from flu and its potentially serious complications. Studies show that flu vaccination reduces the risk of flu illness by 40 to 60 percent among the overall population during flu seasons.

____

____

____

____

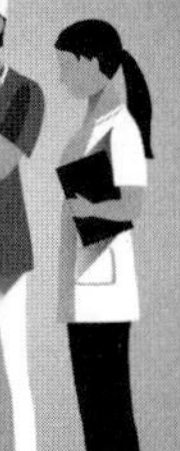

To conclude, flu can be prevented if you are aware of the above tips. Remember that prevention is always the best medicine which can save you from unnecessary suffering.

- To find more information about the prevention of flu, you may refer to the following source.
  CDC. 2023. Preventive steps. Retrieved April 3, 2023, from CDC website.

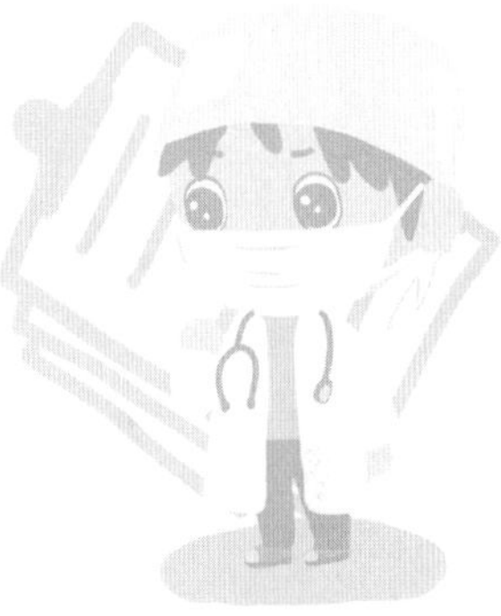

Unit 2
Medicine

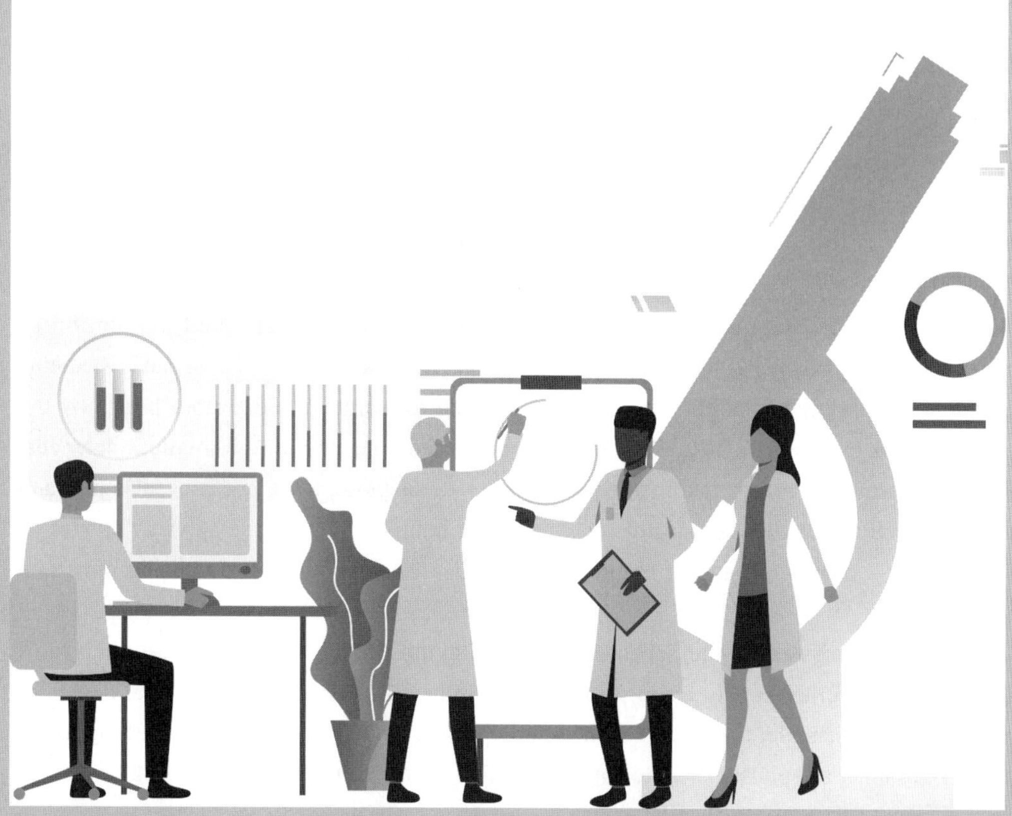

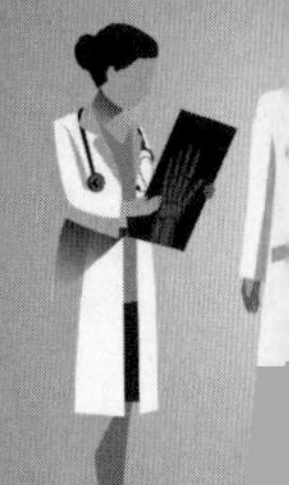

Part A | Information Searching and Delivering

I. Surf on the Internet and find information about the following topics before class.

1. alternative medicine
2. functional diagnosis
3. conventional medicine
4. traditional medicine
5. gene therapy

II. Make a presentation based on the information you've searched.

Part B | Text Understanding

Passage 1 Medicine

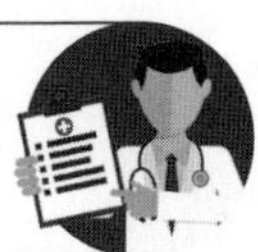

Medicine is the science and practice of the diagnosis, treatment, and prevention of disease. The word "medicine" is derived from Latin *medicus*, meaning "a physician". Medicine encompasses a variety of health care practices evolved to maintain and restore health by the prevention and treatment of illness. Contemporary medicine applies biomedical sciences, biomedical research, genetics, and medical technology to diagnose, treat, and prevent injury and disease, typically through pharmaceuticals or surgery, but also through therapies as diverse as psychotherapy, external splints and traction, medical devices, biologics, and ionizing radiation, amongst others.

Medicine has existed for thousands of years, during most of which it was an art (an area of skill and knowledge) frequently having connections to the religious and philosophical beliefs of local culture. For example, a medicine man would apply herbs and say prayers for healing, or an ancient philosopher and physician would apply bloodletting according to the theories of humorism.

In recent centuries, since the advent of modern science, most medicine has become a combination of art and science (both basic and applied, under the umbrella of medical science). While stitching technique for sutures is an art learned through practice, the knowledge of what happens at the cellular and molecular level in the tissues being stitched arises through science.

Prescientific forms of medicine are now known as traditional medicine and folk medicine. They remain commonly used with or instead of scientific medicine and are thus called alternative medicine. For example, evidence on the effectiveness of acupuncture is "variable and inconsistent" for any condition, but acupuncture is generally safe when done by an appropriately trained practitioner. In contrast, treatments outside the bounds of safety and efficacy are termed quackery.

In modern clinical practice, physicians personally assess patients in order to diagnose, treat, and prevent disease using clinical judgment. The doctor-patient relationship typically begins an interaction with an examination of the patient's medical history and medical record, followed by a medical interview and a physical examination. Basic diagnostic medical devices (e.g. stethoscope, tongue depressor) are typically used. After examination for signs and interviewing for symptoms, the doctor may order medical tests (e.g. blood tests), take a biopsy, or prescribe pharmaceutical drugs or other therapies. Differential diagnosis methods help to rule out conditions based on the information provided. During the encounter, properly informing the patient of all relevant facts is an important part of the relationship and the development of trust. The medical encounter is then documented in the medical record, which is a legal document in many jurisdictions. Follow-ups may be shorter but follow the same general procedure, and specialists follow a similar process. The diagnosis and treatment may take only a few minutes or a few weeks depending upon the complexity of the issue.

Contemporary medicine is in general conducted within health care systems. Legal, credentialing and financing frameworks are established by individual governments, and augmented on occasion by international organizations, such as churches. The characteristics of any given health care system have significant impact on the way medical care is provided.

From ancient times, Christian emphasis on practical charity gave rise to the development of systematic nursing and hospitals and the Catholic Church today remains the largest non-government provider of medical services in the world. Advanced industrial countries and many developing countries provide medical services through a system of universal health care that aims to guarantee care for all through a single-payer health care system, or compulsory private or co-operative health insurance. This is intended to ensure that the entire population has access to medical care on the basis of need rather than ability to pay. Delivery may be via private medical practices or by state-owned hospitals and clinics, or by charities, most commonly by a combination of all three.

Most tribal societies provide no guarantee of healthcare for the population as a whole. In such societies, healthcare is available to those that can afford to pay for it or have self-insured it (either directly or as part of an employment contract) or who may be covered by healthcare financed by the government or tribe directly.

In low-income countries, modern healthcare is often too expensive for the average person. International healthcare policy researchers have advocated that "user fees" be removed in these areas to ensure access, although even after removal, significant costs and barriers remain.

It is generally the goal of most countries to have their health services organized in such a way to ensure that individuals, families, and communities obtain the maximum benefit from current knowledge and technology available for the promotion, maintenance, and restoration of health. In order to play their part in this process, governments and other agencies are still faced with numerous tasks.

Source: Wikipedia and Britannica.

I. Match the words with their definitions according to Passage 1.

Words	Definitions
____ 1. encompass	a limit or boundary
____ 2. advent	b that must be done because of a law or a rule
____ 3. acupuncture	c the process of giving birth to a baby
____ 4. bound	d the coming of an important event, person, invention, etc.
____ 5. efficacy	e the removal and examination of tissue from the body of sb. who is ill, in order to find out more about their disease
____ 6. biopsy	f the ability of sth., especially a drug or a medical treatment, to produce the results that are wanted
____ 7. jurisdiction	g the aim of giving money, food, help, etc. to people who are in need
____ 8. charity	h to include a large number or range of things
____ 9. compulsory	i a Chinese method of treating pain and illness using special thin needles which are pushed into the skin in particular parts of the body
____ 10. delivery	j an area or a country in which a particular system of laws has authority

II. Read Passage 1 and answer the following questions.

1. What's the definition and etymology of medicine?

____

2. What is alternative medicine?

____

3. What does "medical encounter" refer to in Paragraph 4?

____

4. How are medical services delivered to the entire population?

____

5. What is the goal of health service in most countries?

____

Passage 2 What Are the Benefits and Advantages of Telemedicine?

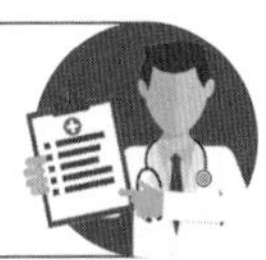

The medical world is constantly changing. Technology now plays a big role in the medical domain. As doctors regularly look for better ways to treat people, technology has brought numerous great advances to the medical field. Thanks to technological advancements such as telemedicine, you can obtain access to medical services or information that might normally be unavailable.

Telemedicine is the exchange of medical information from one site to another through electronic communications. This is done for the purpose of improving a person's health.

Telemedicine has been around for over 40 years. It is a rapidly growing field. It can be very difficult to get an appointment with primary care doctors and specialists. The waiting list can be long, and even getting a referral doesn't guarantee a quick appointment. Telemedicine can help bring you and the doctor together more efficiently.

Depending on your healthcare provider's setup, they can use telemedicine for your consultation. Your doctor can forward diagnostic images such as X-rays and your medical history to the telemedicine doctor for them to review. The telemedicine doctor may have enough information to make a diagnosis and even create the appropriate treatment plan. If not, they can contact you or your doctor for more information. Together you all can decide on the best treatment plan.

Some healthcare professionals have remote patient monitoring systems set up. These remote

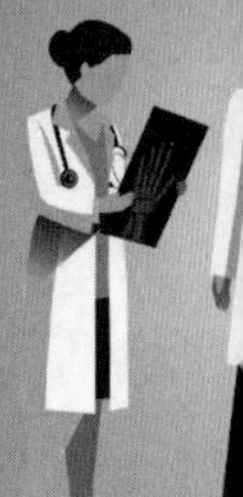

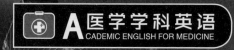

systems are constantly collecting and sending data to other healthcare agencies for interpretation. This is an important step in telemedicine because even if you are homebound, you can easily get your latest health information over to your doctor. A nurse can come, set up all the equipment in your home, conduct the needed tests, and transmit the data to the doctor before the close of business.

Telemedicine is great for doctors and people seeking medical treatment when it comes to treatment and diagnosis. It can also be a great support system. You can use it to get consumer medical and health information from the Internet. For example, if you or a loved one is fighting cancer, you can link up and get specialized information and get involved in online peer discussion groups.

Online peer discussion groups not only provide helpful information, but also, more importantly, support. Meeting other people going through the same thing as you can help you feel less alone. It can be encouraging and offer peace of mind.

Even doctors have to brush up on their skills from time to time, and telemedicine is right there to help. Doctors and other medical professionals can listen to lectures and get demonstrations of the latest technology without leaving their office.

This type of telemedicine technology is even more important for healthcare officials volunteering in distant places or currently serving in the military. Medical facilities are not always nearby. Receiving treatment or information can be almost impossible. Telemedicine can help save a life.

There are several advantages to telemedicine. One of the biggest is it gives you access to specialists and information that you might not readily have access to otherwise. During a telemedicine consultation, you usually have a chance to tell the doctor about your medical history and ask questions. In turn, the specialist can ask you questions directly.

This telemedicine setup is better than trying to relay information to your doctor or nurse, and then having them relay the message. The specialist can hear the sound of your cough or see your swollen eyes. You can hear firsthand about your diagnosis and treatment options. Telemedicine is considered a regular healthcare service. In most cases, it should be billable to your health care insurance without issue.

According to studies, telemedicine may save money, both for the person receiving treatment and for the provider, when compared to traditional care. For this to be true, though, the healthcare facility must have telemedicine equipment on-site. Telemedicine definitely has its strong points, but there are some disadvantages.

One of the main disadvantages is availability and cost. You may not have access to telemedicine services. For the provider, it can be expensive to set up and maintain. Though a great and worthy service, telemedicine may be too costly for smaller healthcare facilities.

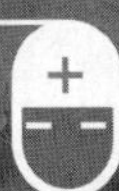

Telemedicine can open up many treatment doors, but it is not the same as a brick-and-mortar doctor office. If you prefer a more personal or face-to-face relationship, telemedicine might not be the option for you. You often do not get a chance to bond with your telemedicine doctor, and you may never get a chance to personally meet them. You may not even get a chance to video conference with the specialist.

Certain types of illnesses and problems require a face-to-face physical assessment and cannot be diagnosed through telemedicine.

Though no service is perfect, telemedicine is a positive and growing medical treatment option. Studies continue to show that telemedicine saves time, money, and lives.

With the rapidly rising cost of healthcare, and the fact that it is nonexistent in some places, the need for telemedicine continues to grow. It may not be the option for everyone, but the pros seem to outweigh the cons. Being able to treat patients from their home, give valuable medical support and information, and provide service to less developed areas makes it hard to pass up.

Source: Wu, B. 2016. What are the benefits and advantages of telemedicine? Retrieved May 16, 2020, from Healthline website.

I. Match the words with their definitions according to Passage 2.

____ 1. domain	ⓐ to watch and check sth. over a period of time in order to see how it develops, so that you can make any necessary changes
____ 2. referral	ⓑ not present under specified conditions or in a specified place
____ 3. forward	ⓒ quickly and without difficulty
____ 4. monitor	ⓓ to develop or create a relationship of trust and affection with sb.
____ 5. readily	ⓔ to receive and send on information, news, etc. to sb.
____ 6. relay	ⓕ an area of knowledge or activity
____ 7. swollen	ⓖ to send or pass goods or information to sb.
____ 8. bond	ⓗ to be greater or more important than sth.
____ 9. nonexistent	ⓘ the act of sending someone to another person or place for treatment
____ 10. outweigh	ⓙ (of a part of the body) larger than normal, especially as a result of a disease or an injury

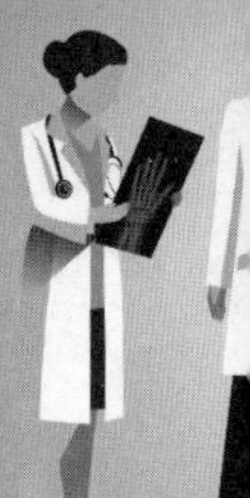

II. Read Passage 2 and answer the following questions.

1. What is telemedicine?

 ____

2. What are the advantages of telemedicine mentioned in the passage?

 ____

3. What does the author mean by saying "it is not the same as a brick-and-mortar doctor office" in the last but three paragraph?

 ____

4. What are the disadvantages of telemedicine mentioned in the passage?

 ____

5. What could be the possible trend of telemedicine?

 ____

Passage 3 Interpreting the Language of Traditional Medicine

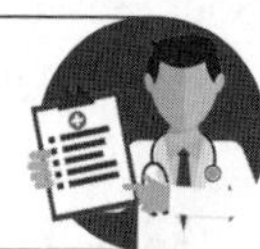

As an academic and clinician who has straddled both the complementary and conventional spaces, it has been relatively easy to grasp the alignment of integrative medicine with broader public health approaches—it is even a topic I have published on in detail. However, such alignment is not always obvious to others, and in some cases this can lead to people suggesting that integrative medicine is somehow incongruent with broader health aims. One reason why this argument often gains currency is the strange language sometimes used by integrative medicine—often derided by critics as being pseudoscientific.

It is undeniable that many terms used in integrative medicine—particularly those aspects drawn from traditional medicine—do sound strange to Western ears. Bodily systems become damp, the vital force becomes weakened, and the essence of certain organs needs to become better tonified. It is no exaggeration to suggest that the language of traditional medicine systems is often far removed from that of biomedicine. However, rather than using linguistic differences to dismiss the value of traditional medicine approaches, these linguistic differences should be examined in further detail to see what they can teach us about health. We don't judge the validity of scientific ideas differently depending on whether they are presented in Swedish, Sinhalese, Swahili or English, and our approach to the various languages of medicine should be no different.

However, this is not what happens in the real world, where politics, ideologies and personal and professional interests often intersect and clash. For example, when the Australian Therapeutic

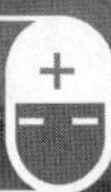

Goods Administration developed a list of allowable traditional medicine claims, critics immediately derided the move, pouncing on the ridiculousness of terms like “tonifies kidney essence” or “softens hardness” as being indicative of the pseudoscientific nature of traditional medicine systems. However, although the terms may sound funny to a Western ear, this represents a linguistic difference rather than an incongruity with science. Indeed, when the terminology of traditional systems like Chinese medicine are examined by linguists, they appear to represent physiological concepts that are recognized in conventional functional diagnoses, but simply represent them in a linguistically different way.

Yet critics often get stuck on the “floral” language often present in traditional medicine terminology and limit their critique to this superficial and overly simplistic interpretation. In doing so they miss the forest for the trees. *Qi* is not a physiological manifestation of white light traversing the body—as is often portrayed in some of the harsher criticisms of Chinese medicine—but rather a conceptual tool that is used to explain functional variations in body systems. Use of such functional diagnoses, conceptual tools and even funny names is not unique to traditional medicine. They are common in conventional medicine, and some functional diagnoses—polycystic ovarian syndrome for example—can be present even without the physiological identifiers that define their very name being present. Is this that different to the use of conceptual organs in traditional medicine systems?

Irritable bowel syndrome—in critic’s mind—is a term at least as non-medical or ridiculous sounding as anything in Chinese medicine, yet it is considered acceptable in conventional medicine. Moreover, as a functional diagnosis, it shares as much of its diagnosis to physiology as a traditional medicine diagnosis. It has even been formulated the same way—by long-term expert consensus (the Rome Criteria) which has codified symptoms and attributes that relate to the diagnosis. If we are going to argue the validity of traditional medicine diagnoses because they are functional or conceptual rather than physiological, we also need to examine the validity of those used in conventional practice.

And these are not unusual examples. The fields of psychiatry and psychology are almost entirely dependent on conceptual and functional diagnoses of the Diagnostic Statistical Manual (DSM). Whilst admittedly the DSM (and to some degree psychiatry and psychology) has come under some criticism recently, this is qualitatively different from the criticism faced by integrative medicine. Whilst the very existence of traditional medicine texts is questioned, the critique of the DSM is directed at the over-reach and industry influence of some diagnoses, rather than whether the tool itself or the manner in which it has been developed was in-and-of itself valid.

The false dichotomy that is often presented between conventional and complementary medicine can explain some of these differences. We are told that if a complementary medicine worked it would simply become conventional medicine, but the truth is far more complex than that, with multiple examples of conventional treatments continuing to be used after we know

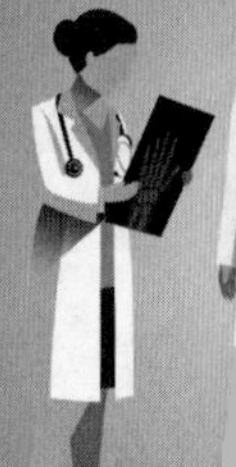

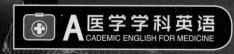

they do not work, and multiple complementary treatments still not integrated even when they do. We are told that complementary medicine promotes the rejection of conventional medicine (for example rejection of vaccination or cancer treatment), when the truth is far more complicated than that (for example, there is more support than opposition for vaccination in the complementary medicine community). Complementary medicine criticism often attracts lazy arguments, built on assumptions rather than facts, and the superficial dismissal of the different languages used by traditional medicine is an extension of this.

However, it need not be this way. Indeed, it should not be this way. As clinicians and researchers aspiring for the best for our patients, we should be viewing all systems and languages of medicine objectively to see what we can learn for the promotion of better health for all. At *Advances* we are increasingly seeing submissions that are based on traditional medicine diagnosis. Initially we were hesitant to publish them based solely on the notion that a broad readership may not be fluent on the languages of certain traditions; but we are increasingly embracing them so that clinicians can become multi-lingual in the various languages of health. We hope that this will be a fruitful—if challenging—learning experience for all of us, as we become familiar with new ways of talking about health and explore what does and does not work best for patients.

This is not to say that we should not be critical of some elements of traditional practice—indeed, de-implementation of practices that are ineffective or harmful is just as important as implementation of practices that are useful—but it does suggest we need to be more open as to where we seek information. This necessitates looking beyond the limited language of biomedicine or narrowly focusing on single traditions of practice—and highlights the importance of drawing on wisdom from multiple healing traditions and approaches.

Source: Wardle, J. 2019. Interpreting the language of traditional medicine. *Advances in Integrative Medicine, 6:* 93-94.

I. Match the words with their definitions according to Passage 3.

____ 1. deride	ⓐ an opinion that all members of a group agree with
____ 2. pseudoscientific	ⓑ to move to and fro over
____ 3. fruitful	ⓒ a quality or characteristic inherent in or ascribed to someone or something
____ 4. traverse	ⓓ to treat sb./sth. as ridiculous and not worth considering seriously
____ 5. ovarian	ⓔ the separation that exists between two groups or things that are completely opposite to and different from each other

____ 6. consensus	f	using or having the ability to use several languages
____ 7. attribute	g	the act of giving a document, proposal, etc. to sb. in authority so that they can study or consider it
____ 8. dichotomy	h	of or relating to an ovary
____ 9. submission	i	producing many useful results
____ 10. multi-lingual	j	based on theories and methods erroneously regarded as scientific

II. Read Passage 3 and answer the following questions.

1. What is the profession of the author according to the passage?
____

2. How do you understand "In doing so they miss the forest for the trees" (Paragraph 4)?
____

3. Why integrative medicine is inconsistent with broader health aims?
____

4. Why does the author mention the attitude change of *Advances*?
____

5. What's the author's attitude toward the elements of traditional practice?
____

III. Read the three passages comprehensively and answer the following questions.

1. What is the common theme of the three passages?
____

2. What are the differences among the three passages in terms of topic?
____

3. What's your opinion on conventional medicine and traditional medicine?
____

4. Write a short passage of about 100 words to synthesize the information of the three passages.
____
____
____
____
____

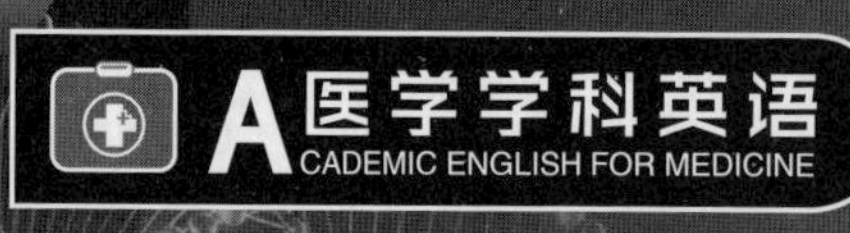

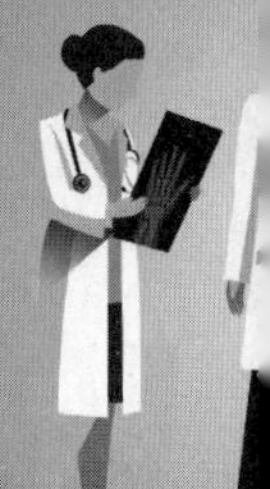

Part C Integrated Exercises

I. Read the words below, and pay attention to the pronunciation. Use the scale below (1, 2, 3) to give yourself a score for each word. Try to consult your dictionary for the words with score 1.

❶ I don't understand this word.

❷ I understand this word when I see it or hear it, but I don't know how to use it.

❸ I know this word and can use it in my own speaking and writing.

Academic words

□ advent	□ advocate	□ alignment	□ aspire
□ attribute	□ augment	□ billable	□ bound
□ codify	□ complementary	□ complexity	□ compulsory
□ consensus	□ consultation	□ contemporary	□ conventional
□ credential	□ currency	□ deride	□ dichotomy
□ differential	□ dismiss	□ document	□ domain
□ effectiveness	□ efficacy	□ embrace	□ encompass
□ encounter	□ evolve	□ external	□ formulate
□ forward	□ framework	□ harsh	□ identifier
□ incongruent	□ inconsistent	□ integrative	□ intersect
□ jurisdiction	□ maintenance	□ manifestation	□ multi-lingual
□ necessitate	□ outweigh	□ quackery	□ qualitatively
□ readership	□ readily	□ referral	□ restoration
□ seek	□ simplistic	□ statistical	□ straddle
□ submission	□ superficial	□ systematic	□ validity

Discipline-specific words

□ acupuncture	□ biologics	□ biomedical	□ biomedicine
□ biopsy	□ bloodletting	□ cellular	□ clinician
□ cough	□ depressor	□ diagnosis	□ healthcare

☐ herb	☐ humorism	☐ medical	☐ molecular
☐ organ	☐ ovarian	☐ pharmaceutical	☐ physician
☐ physiological	☐ poly-cystic	☐ practitioner	☐ prescribe
☐ provider	☐ psychiatry	☐ psychotherapy	☐ *Qi*
☐ radiation	☐ rejection	☐ splint	☐ stethoscope
☐ suture	☐ swollen	☐ syndrome	☐ telemedicine
☐ therapeutic	☐ therapy	☐ tissue	☐ tonify
☐ traction	☐ treatment	☐ vaccination	

II. Match each word in the box with the group of words that regularly occur in academic writing.

maintain	establish	augment	formulate	seek
embrace	advocate	codify	dismiss	transmit

1. ____________ disease / virus / data / a message
2. ____________ an idea / technology / a change
3. ____________ income / power / capability
4. ____________ treatment / advice / help / refuge
5. ____________ law / an act / a rule
6. ____________ an employee / an appeal / the case
7. ____________ reform / right / an approach
8. ____________ a school / a relationship / reputation / a system
9. ____________ health / balance / quality
10. ____________ a plan / a hypothesis / a strategy

III. Study the members of the word families in the table below. Try to work out the meaning in each case according to its prefix or suffix.

The members of a word family	Chinese definitions
prescribe, prescriber, prescription, prescriptive	开（处方）、开处方者、处方、指定的
vary, variable, variant, variation, variance	
radiate, radiative, radiation	

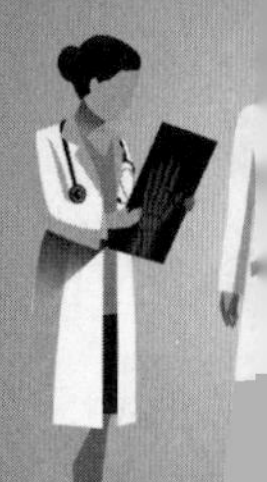

restore, restorable, restoration	
therapy, therapist, therapeutic	
specialize, specialization, specialist, specialty	
biology, biological, biologist, biologics	
clinic, clinical, clinician	
medicine, medicinal, medicinally	
incongruent, incongruity, incongruently	
physiology, physiological, physiologically, physiologist	
necessary, necessitate, necessity	
critic, critique, critical, criticize	
integrate, integrative, integration	
consult, consultant, consultation	
valid, validate, validity	
simple, simplify, simplification, simplistic	
psychology, psychological, psychologist, psychotherapy, psychosis, psychiatry	
complement, complementary, complementation	

IV. Complete each sentence below with a word from the table above.

1. Antibiotics are only available on ________. (prescribe)
2. The paper says at least 10 people have been killed by a ________ of the strain known as adenovirus 14. (vary)
3. Overall, women who did not complete ________ had a slightly higher risk of a cancer recurrence over the next 5 years. (radiate)
4. Our ________ style offers release from stored tensions, traumas, and grief. (therapy)
5. Her family members do not have similar ________ manifestations. Her mother had been dead for unknown etiological factors. (clinic)

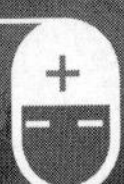

6. A couple of recent medical studies had suggested that running long distances might be ________ damaging. (physiology)
7. His other injuries have healed remarkably well, and no longer ________ any special care. (necessary)
8. Their ________ medical approach will appeal to readers who want to be well-informed about all their options. (integrate)
9. ________ explanations, such as blaming obesity on a drop-in fat consumption, ignore scientific reality. (simple)
10. Such a treatment exploits the ________ action of two or more antibiotics. (complement)

V. Choose the word in each list that is not a synonym for the underlined word.

1. <u>diverse</u>

   A. varied B. identical C. disparate D. dissimilar
2. <u>external</u>

   A. internal B. outer C. extrinsic D. exterior
3. <u>inconsistent</u>

   A. conflicting B. discrepant C. incompatible D. congruent
4. <u>complexity</u>

   A. complication B. simplicity C. sophistication D. intricacy
5. <u>admittedly</u>

   A. confessedly B. avowedly C. denyingly D. acknowledgedly
6. <u>conventional</u>

   A. traditional B. customary C. ordinary D. revolutionary
7. <u>overly</u>

   A. insufficiently B. excessively C. exceedingly D. unduly
8. <u>portray</u>

   A. depict B. describe C. distort D. delineate
9. <u>implementation</u>

   A. application B. dismissal C. execution D. enforcement
10. <u>barrier</u>

    A. hindrance B. obstacle C. aid D. impediment

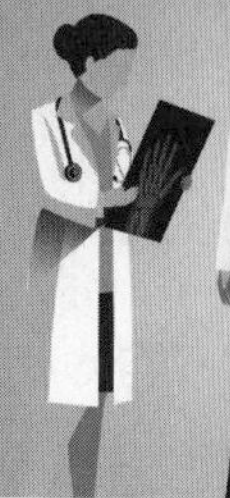

VI. Read the following expressions and sentence patterns aloud and analyze the formality of the structures used.

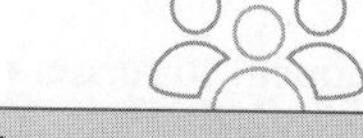

Target sentence patterns

1. Contemporary medicine **applies** biomedical sciences, biomedical research, genetics, and medical technology **to** diagnose, treat, and prevent injury and disease, typically **through** pharmaceuticals or surgery, but also through therapies **as** diverse **as** psychotherapy, external splints and traction, medical devices, biologics, and ionizing radiation, **amongst others**.
2. In recent centuries, **since the advent of** modern science, most medicine has become **a combination of** art and science (both basic and applied, **under the umbrella of** medical science).
3. Differential diagnosis methods help to **rule out** conditions based on the information provided.
4. From ancient times, Christian **emphasis on** practical charity **gave rise to** the development of systematic nursing and hospitals and the Catholic Church today remains the largest non-government provider of medical services in the world.
5. This is **intended to** ensure that the entire population **has access to** medical care **on the basis of** need **rather than** ability to pay.
6. In order to **play their part in** this process, governments and other agencies **are** still **faced with** numerous tasks.
7. Advanced industrial countries and many developing countries provide medical services through a system of universal health care **that aims to** guarantee care for all through a single-payer health care system, or compulsory private or co-operative health insurance.
8. **However**, such alignment is not always **obvious to** others, and **in some cases** this can **lead to** people suggesting **that** integrative medicine **is** somehow **incongruent with** broader health aims.
9. **It is undeniable that** many terms used in integrative medicine—particularly those aspects drawn from traditional medicine—do sound strange to Western ears.
10. **It is no exaggeration to** suggest that the language of traditional medicine systems is often far removed from that of biomedicine.
11. Yet critics often **get stuck on** the "floral" language often present in traditional medicine terminology and limit their critique to this superficial and overly simplistic interpretation.
12. As clinicians and researchers **aspiring for** the best for our patients, we should be viewing all systems and languages of medicine objectively to see what we can learn for the promotion of

better health for all.

13. Initially we **were hesitant to** publish them based solely on the notion that a broad readership may not be fluent on the languages of certain traditions;
14. One reason why this argument often **gains currency** is the strange language sometimes used by integrative medicine—often derided by critics as being pseudoscientific.
15. *Qi* is not a physiological **manifestation of** white light traversing the body—**as** is often portrayed in some of the harsher criticisms of Chinese medicine—**but rather** a conceptual tool that is used to explain functional variations in body systems.
16. The fields of psychiatry and psychology **are** almost entirely **dependent on** conceptual and functional diagnoses of the Diagnostic Statistical Manual (DSM).
17. **Whilst** admittedly the DSM (and to some degree psychiatry and psychology) has come **under some criticism** recently, this is qualitatively different from the criticism faced by integrative medicine.
18. Complementary medicine criticism often **attracts** lazy **arguments**, built on assumptions **rather than** facts, and the superficial dismissal of the different languages used by traditional medicine is **an extension of** this.
19. This is not to say that we should not **be critical of** some elements of traditional practice—indeed, de-implementation of practices that are ineffective or harmful is just **as** important **as** implementation of practices that are useful—**but** it does suggest we need to be more open as to where we seek information.
20. **In doing so** they miss the forest for the trees.
21. **Thanks to** technological advancements such as telemedicine, you can **obtain access to** medical services or information that might normally be unavailable.
22. If you or a loved one is fighting cancer, you can **link up** and get specialized information and **get involved in** online peer discussion groups.
23. Even doctors have to **brush up on** their skills from time to time, and telemedicine is right there to help.
24. It may not be the option for everyone, but **the pros seem to outweigh the cons.**
25. **According to** studies, telemedicine may save money, both for the person receiving treatment and for the provider, when **compared to** traditional care.

VII. For each of the sentences below, write a new sentence as similar as possible in meaning to the original one, but as formal as possible in style.

1. Most importantly, we'd recommend consulting a medical practitioner or dietitian before refusing any major food group like dairy from the diet.

2. Therapeutic Drug Monitoring <u>is used to</u> optimize drug therapy by knowing the measured concentration and therapeutic effect.

3. This isn't different from a low-fat diet, <u>except</u> that a low-fat diet is used for weight loss.

4. <u>Everyone knows the fact that</u> a person who is having a sensitive skin must have a dry texture.

5. <u>It is not too much to say</u> that modern Americans cannot survive the life in which there are no products made in China.

6. Traditional Chinese medicine <u>becomes popular</u> in Lebanon.

7. <u>We cannot say</u> the object <u>depends on</u> the perception of a single mind.

8. Freud <u>was</u> severely <u>criticized</u> for <u>advocating</u> the drug.

9. This kind of discretion also <u>caused discussions</u> on traditional Chinese medical science.

10. Blood donation <u>does more good than harm</u>, so it should be encouraged under scientific instructions.

VIII. Translate the following sentences by using the following words and phrases. Make sure that your English sentences are different from the Chinese versions in terms of structures or orders, but as formal as possible. Then compare yours with your partner's according to the criteria: Whose version is more different and more formal?

1. 可以将这一类似的技术应用于癌症的治疗。(apply to)

____

2. 该国的血库均属于红十字会。(under the umbrella of)

____

3. 体内胆碱水平过低会引起高血压。(give rise to)

____

4. 大麻作为药物仍然受到该国医生的抵制。(be faced with)

____

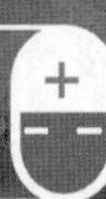

5. 新发现可能会实现对帕金森氏病的有效自然治疗。(lead to)

____

6. 医师似乎不愿强制中断癌症治疗。(be hesitant to)

____

7. 我无意批评这些医学试验，只是它们不足以回答这一问题。(be critical of)

____

8. 多亏近年来的研究，才有了有效的疗法。(thanks to)

____

9. 无论发生什么情况，他们和他们的家人都能够获得抗病毒药物。(obtain access to)

____

10. 你可以有多种方式去参与世界卫生组织工作。(get involved in)

____

Part D Academic Skills

Academic Listening Skill

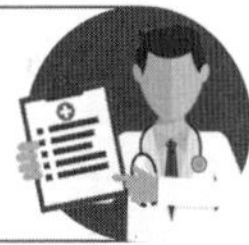

Recognizing Signal Words

While listening, you may find it's difficult to follow the speaker's ideas. However, the speaker will use specific words and phrases called signal words to help you follow his/her organization. These words act as markers or sign posts that indicate what kind of information the speaker will give next. They can be used for many different purposes. When you can grasp them, you can predict what will come next, and as a result, your notes will be more complete and accurate. Here are some examples of commonly used signal words:

To signal a new idea: now...; let me start with...; next, let's talk about...

To signal a definition: that is, ...; in other words, ...; X, meaning...; the definition of that is...

To signal an example: for example, ...; for instance, ...; ..., such as...

To signal an opposite idea: but; however; on the other hand

To signal causes or effects: so; due to; because of

...

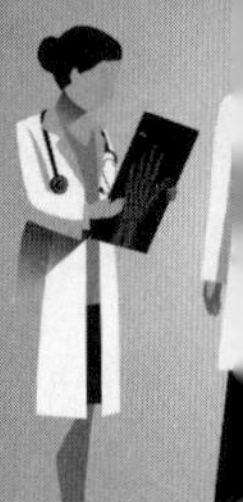

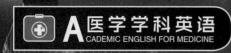

Listening 1

Word bank

1. anatomy	the scientific study of the structure of human or animal bodies
2. physiology	the scientific study of the normal functions of living things
3. biochemistry	the scientific study of the chemistry of living things
4. pharmacology	the scientific study of drugs and their use in medicine
5. pathology	the scientific study of diseases
6. diagnose	to say exactly what an illness or the cause of a problem is
7. defective	having a fault or faults; not perfect or complete
8. stethoscope	an instrument that a doctor uses to listen to sb's heart and breathing
9. genuine	real; exactly what it appears to be
10. practitioner	a person who works in a profession, especially medicine or law
11. neurology	the scientific study of nerves and their diseases
12. orthopedic	marked by or affected with a skeletal deformity, disorder, or injury
13. cardiovascular	pertaining to the heart and blood vessels
14. titanium	a light strong white metal
15. psychiatrist	a doctor who studies and treats mental illnesses

I. Listen to the passage and choose the best answer to each of the questions.

1 What does the passage mainly talk about?

A The job of a general practitioner.

B How to become a qualified doctor.

C Introduction to the job and the classifications of doctors.

D The differences between a psychiatrist and a hospital doctor.

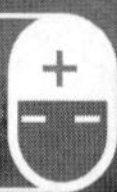

❷ **Which one of the following options is NOT the duty of a hospital doctor?**

Ⓐ Detecting bowel cancer.

Ⓑ Providing routine checkups.

Ⓒ Fulfilling emergency medicine.

Ⓓ Putting titanium plates in the patient's body.

❸ **What can a cardiologist do?**

Ⓐ A cardiologist can deal with patient mental health conditions which impair day-to-day functions.

Ⓑ A cardiologist can deal with the diagnosis and treatment of diseases and disorders of the heart.

Ⓒ A cardiologist corrects abnormalities of bones such as putting titanium plates in patients so they can walk again.

Ⓓ A cardiologist provides routine checkups, diagnosing, assessing, and treating hundreds of conditions.

II. Tick the signal words appearing in this listening material. And then classify them with A to F according to their different functions.

Ⓐ showing the results	Ⓑ stressing
Ⓒ classification	Ⓓ further illustration
Ⓔ transition	Ⓕ giving examples

1. well	( ) ________	2. moreover	( ) ________
3. again	( ) ________	4. in other words	( ) ________
5. for instance	( ) ________	6. finally	( ) ________
7. for example	( ) ________	8. due to	( ) ________
9. first of all	( ) ________	10. even if	( ) ________
11. so	( ) ________	12. now that	( ) ________
13. let's talk	( ) ________	14. just remember that	( ) ________

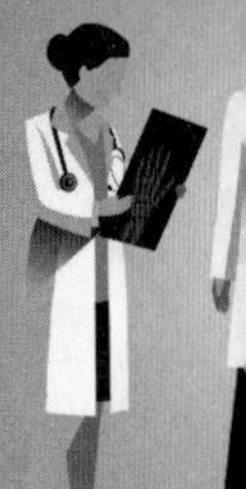

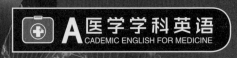

Listening 2 

Word bank

1. lining	the covering of the inner surface of a part of the body
2. intestine	a long tube in the body between the stomach and the anus
3. acid	a chemical, usually a liquid, that contains hydrogen and has a PH of less than seven
4. bile	a yellow or greenish viscid alkaline fluid secreted by the liver and passed into the duodenum where it aids especially in the emulsification and absorption of fats
5. bruise	an injury involving rupture of small blood vessels and discoloration without a break in the overlying skin
6. skeleton	the structure of bones that supports the body of a person or an animal
7. neuron	a cell that carries information within the brain and between the brain and other parts of the body
8. circuit	a neuronal pathway of the brain along which electrical and chemical signals travel
9. cluster	a group of things of the same type that grow or appear close together
10. transparent	allowing light to pass through so that objects behind can be distinctly seen
11. protein	a natural substance found in meat, eggs, fish and some vegetables
12. beat up	give a beating to

Listen to the passage and take notes while listening. Then complete the following exercises. 

Unit 2 Medicine

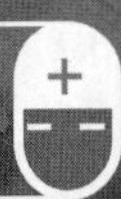

I. Listen to the passage and choose the best answer to each of the following questions.

❶ How often are your muscles refreshed?

Ⓐ Every day.

Ⓑ Every year.

Ⓒ Every 2 to 7 years.

Ⓓ Every 15 years.

❷ Which one of the following options is NOT true?

Ⓐ Each hair on your head is replaced every 2 to 7 years.

Ⓑ Fingernails are completely new every six months or so.

Ⓒ Cells of your heart are replaced every 5 years.

Ⓓ Almost every part of your body refreshes itself.

II. Listen to the passage again and fill in the blanks. Pay attention to the signal words which have been italicized.

1. *I'm not just talking about* the style. Each hair on your head is ________ every ________ to ________ years.
2. *It turns out* it's just a matter of time before almost every part of your body ______________ in a ______________.
3. *And so* those ________ get replaced every few days.
4. *Every few weeks*, your outer layer of skin is completely________.
5. It's *actually* the ________ products of these red blood cells that turn your bruises and urine yellow.
6. You might think you gain and lose fat cells when you gain and lose weight, *but* they *actually* just get ________ and ________.
7. About half of your heart stays with you from birth to death *because* those ______________ ______________.

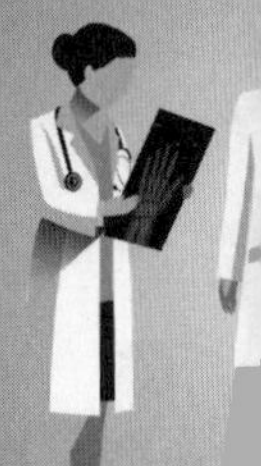

Academic Reading Skill

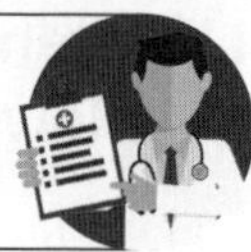

Skimming and Scanning

Skimming and scanning are two important reading strategies which can make reading economical, that is, to read less for the same gain. Skimming is a fast reading method to help readers understand the general theme and general meaning of a passage and paragraph. Skimming prepares readers to deal with the following 4 tasks: summarizing texts, finding main points, restating the subject and giving a suitable title to the text. To skim, you should:

1. pay attention to indicators like *titles, heading, subheading, boldface or italicized words and phrases*, *numerals* like *(1), (2), (3),* or *signals*. Signals include bullets and numbering like *a, b, c,* •, √, or sequencing words or phrases, like *first, second, to begin, to start with*, or words and phrases used to shift the topic like *back to, in regard to, with regard to*.
2. read the first and last paragraph to grasp the subject matter.
3. read the first sentence of each paragraph to grasp researchers' stance or the main idea of each paragraph.
4. look at the diagrams with captions.

Unlike skimming, scanning is search-reading or focused reading. It means that you intentionally search for specific details and fix your attention on certain information while ignoring those irrelevant one. To scan, you should:

1. keep in mind the required information.
2. move eyes down rapidly until you spot the information you are looking for.
3. carefully read the part that contains the required information.

I. Choose the best answer in the following sentence.

If the reader wants to search for specific information in the text, he/she uses ________; if the reader wants to grasp the main idea of the passage, he/she uses ________________.

Ⓐ skimming

Ⓑ scanning

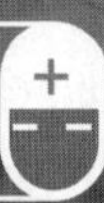

II. Skim the following extracts and choose the best answer to the question.

❶ Prescientific forms of medicine are now known as traditional medicine and folk medicine. They remain commonly used with or instead of scientific medicine and are thus called alternative medicine. For example, evidence on the effectiveness of acupuncture is "variable and inconsistent" for any condition, but is generally safe when done by an appropriately trained practitioner. In contrast, treatments outside the bounds of safety and efficacy are termed quackery.

➢ **What is the main idea of this paragraph?**

Ⓐ Traditional medicine is quackery.

Ⓑ Acupuncture belongs to alternative medicine.

Ⓒ The criterion for distinguishing alternative medicine from quackery is effectiveness.

Ⓓ Once practiced by qualified doctors, traditional medicine and folk medicine is called alternative medicine and it can be used with or instead of scientific medicine.

❷ Functional Medicine is a systems biology-based approach that focuses on identifying and addressing the root cause of disease. Each symptom or differential diagnosis may be one of many contributing factors to an individual's illness.

A diagnosis can be the result of more than one cause. For example, depression can be caused by many different factors, including inflammation. Likewise, a cause such as inflammation may lead to a number of different diagnoses, including depression. The precise manifestation of each cause depends on the individual's genes, environment, and lifestyle, and only treatments that address the right cause will have lasting benefits beyond symptom suppression.

➢ **Which statement is NOT mentioned in the passage?**

Ⓐ Functional medicine attaches importance to identifying and approaching the root cause of disease.

Ⓑ One cause can lead to more than one condition.

Ⓒ A diagnosis must be the result of more than one cause.

Ⓓ The cause of depression can be inflammation.

❸ Telemedicine uses telecommunication and information technology to deliver health care from a distance. Telemedicine has empowered patients in remote areas by enabling them to have health care in their areas.

Telemedicine can also save lives and provide critical care in emergency situations. The technology allows communication between patients and medical staff, as well as the transmission of medical records, images, and other data to and from a remote location.

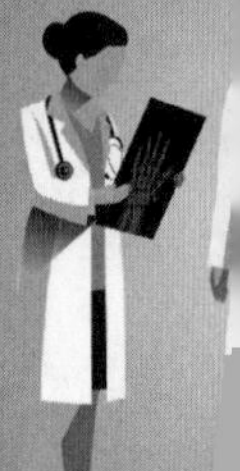

Patients in remote communities can now receive care from doctors including specialists without having to travel long distances at great expense to visit them.

There can even be discussion and collaboration between multiple doctors as if they had all met together. Telemedicine can also be used in medical education by allowing others to observe experts in their field.

➤ **Which of the following is NOT mentioned in this passage?**

Ⓐ Telemedicine delivers health care from a distance by using telecommunication and information technology.

Ⓑ People prefer having telemedicine to having face-to-face communication with doctors.

Ⓒ Telemedicine benefits patients, doctors and medical students in different ways.

Ⓓ Telemedicine is helpful in saving people's lives.

III. Passage 3 states that judging traditional medicine by its language is unreasonable. Hence the language of traditional medicine like *Qi* features in the passage. The author unfolds the passage by showing critics' interpretations of certain language and presenting his own interpretations. Find the traditional medicine language and their interpretations in the passage, and then fill them in the table below. The first example has been given to you.

	Language of traditional medicine	Critics' interpretation	Author's interpretation
1	Bodily systems become damp, ____________, and ____________.	They dismiss the value of traditional medicine approaches by using linguistic difference.	These linguistic differences should be examined in further detail to see what they can teach us about health.
2			
3			
4			

➤ To find more information about how to skim and scan a passage or a paragraph, you may refer to the following sources.

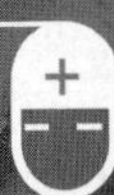

1. Shafiq, M. 2019. What are reading skills? Retrieved May 16, 2020, from Learn Cybers website.
2. Thomas, A. 2017. Reading: Approaching academic texts. Retrieved May 16, 2020, from the University of Edinburgh website.
3. Gillett, A. 2023. Reading skills for academic study. Retrieved May 16, 2020, from UEFAP website.

Academic Writing Skill

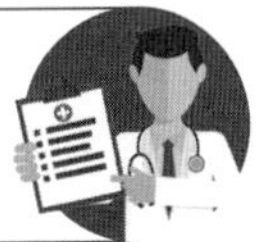

How to Write Definitions

The word definition originates from Latin *definitionem*, which means "a boundary; a limiting, prescribing; an explanation". A definition is a statement of the meaning of a term (a word, phrase, or other set of symbols), expressing the essential nature of something with the help of boundaries or limits. For example, in Passage 1, the author defines medicine as "the science and practice of the diagnosis, treatment, and prevention of disease", expressing the nature of medicine *(science and practice)* with the help of boundaries or limits *(of the diagnosis, treatment, and prevention of disease)*.

In academic writing, it is often necessary to define terms in a formal way, and a formal definition typically consists of three elements:

1. the **term** (word or phrase) to be defined.
2. the **class** to which the term belongs.
3. the **distinguishing detail** that distinguishes it from other terms of the class.

Hence, the structure can be illustrated as follows:

Term + is / is defined as / refers to… + Class + Distinguishing detail

For example: Physiology ***(term)*** is a branch of biology ***(class)*** that deals with the normal functions of living organisms and their parts ***(distinguishing detail)***. The definition gives us a clear statement about the class that diagnosis belongs to and how it is different from other members of the class.

Among the three mentioned elements, distinguishing detail sets the main boundaries or limits for a definition. When writing a distinguishing detail, it is often helpful to use a restrictive relative clause which includes:

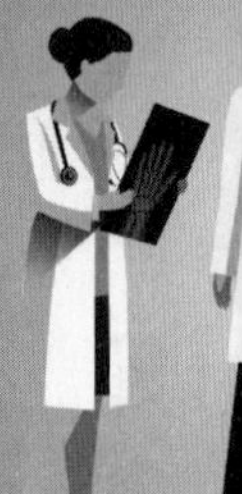

1. **full relative clause** (marked by a relative pronoun such as *that, which* and *who*)
   (Please note: it is not possible to reduce a relative clause if it opens with a preposition)
   - *Acidosis is a condition <u>in which</u> there is too much carbon dioxide in the blood.*
2. **reduced relative clause** (not marked by an explicit relative pronoun)
   a) reduce to a prepositional phrase:
      (Tip: remove the relative pronoun and the verb BE)
      - *Enamel is a hard, white inorganic material (~~that is~~) on the crown of a tooth.*

   b) reduce to a past participle phrase:
      (Tip: remove the relative pronoun and the verb BE)
      - *Osteoporosis is a disease (~~which is~~) characterized by low bone mass and structural deterioration of bone tissue.*

   c) reduce to a present participle phrase:
      (Tip: remove the relative pronoun and change the verb to the -ing form)
      - *Hypertrophy is the enlargement of an organ or part (~~which results~~) resulting from an increase in the size of the cells.*

I. Fill in the blanks with the corresponding elements of the following definitions.

1. Telemedicine is the exchange of medical information from one site to another through electronic communication.
2. Oncology is a branch of medicine concerned with the prevention, diagnosis, treatment, and study of tumor.
3. Hepatitis is an inflammation of the liver that results from a variety of infectious or noninfectious causes.
4. An ophthalmologist is a doctor who specializes in the diagnosis and treatment of diseases of the eye.
5. Bone-remodeling is a process in which old bone tissues are replaced by new bone tissues.

	Term	Class	Distinguishing detail
1			
2			
3			
4			
5			

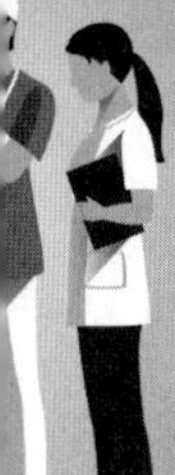

II. Simplify the following definitions by reducing the relative clauses where possible.

1. Tuberculosis is an infectious lung disease which is caused by Mycobacterium tuberculosis.

____

2. Antigen is a kind of substance which causes the formation in the blood of another substance, antibody.

____

3. Neurotransmitter is a chemical by which a nerve cell communicates with another nerve cell or with a muscle.

____

III. Write definitions according to the given elements.

1. Obstetrics—medicine—pregnancy, childbirth, and the postpartum period

____

2. Neurologist—doctor—diagnosis and treatment of diseases of the nervous system

____

3. Asthma—respiratory disorder—difficulty in breathing, wheezing, and a sense of constriction in the chest

____

4. Comminuted fracture—fracture—bone is splintered or crushed

____

5. Basement membrane—layer of connective tissue—epithelium of many organs

____

IV. Now write a definition of a medical term (subject, condition, disease, organ or tissue, etc.) based on the writing skill we've learned.

____

____

____

____

____

____

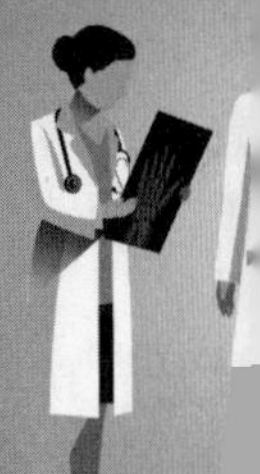

- To find more information about how to write definitions, you may refer to the following source.

  Unified Compliance Framework. 2020. The Definitions Book: How to write definitions. Retrieved August 19, 2020, from Unified Compliance Framework website.

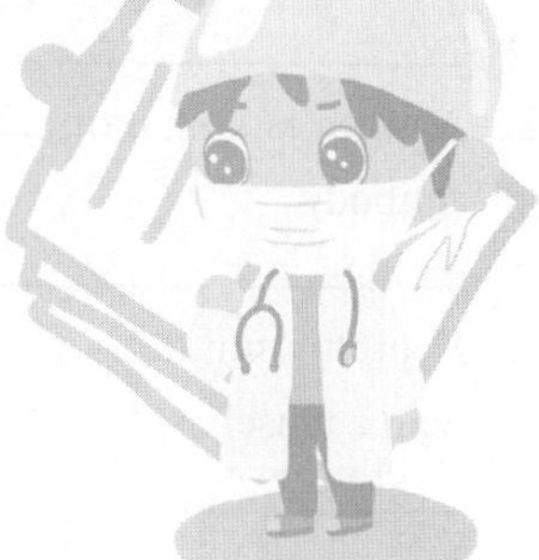

Unit 3

Nursing

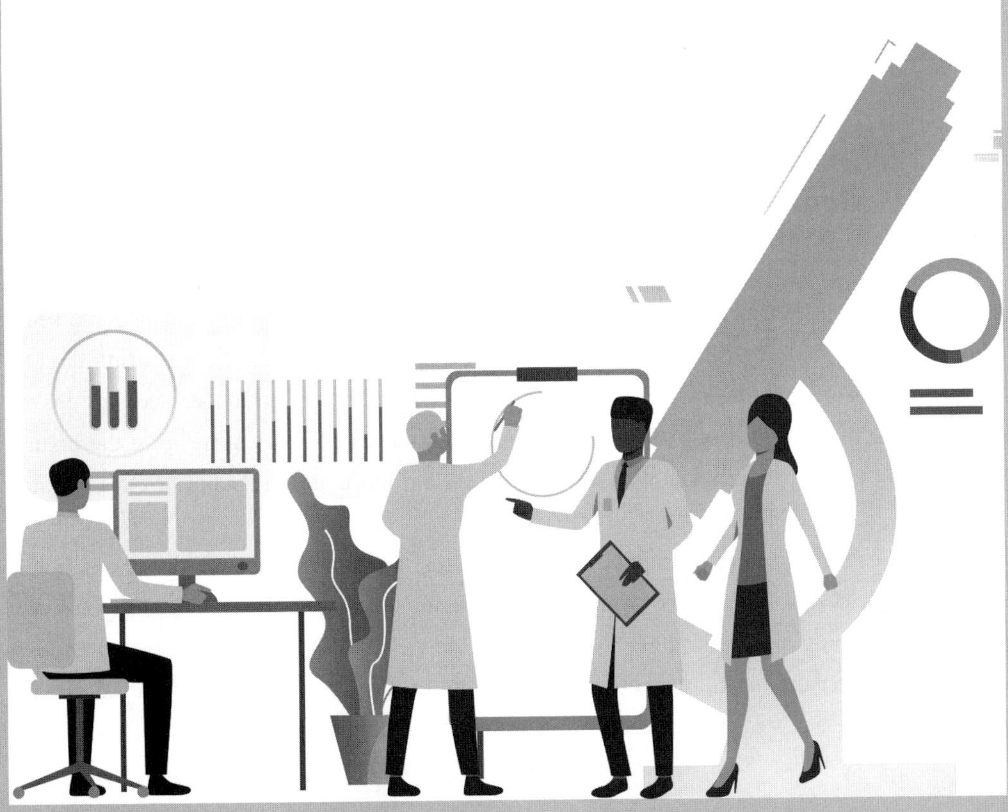

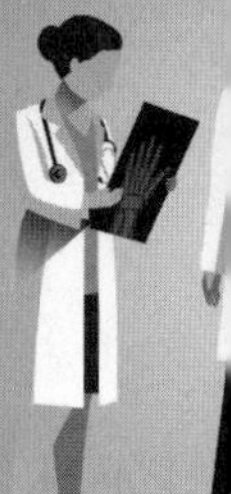

Part A Information Searching and Delivering

I. Surf on the Internet and find information about the following topics before class.

1. Florence Nightingale
2. International Nurses' Day
3. RN (registered nurse)
4. midwife
5. UHC (universal health coverage)

II. Make a presentation based on the information you've searched.

Part B Text Understanding

Passage 1 Men in Nursing: The Challenges in Caregiving

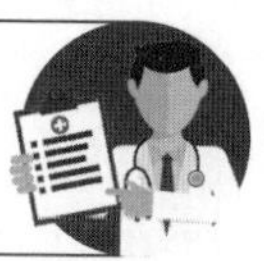

The idea of a male caregiver has been a strange concept for as long as humans have been around. After all, men are the hunters, the providers, and women are the nurturers, right? Evolutionarily this may be the case, but as we evolve even further, we no longer need to rely on biological relics of thousands of years ago. Instead, as an advanced species, we have the luxury of making our own proper decisions that are best for us, our lives, and the people we care about, regardless of what our DNA might say.

It hasn't been until recent years that it's become more acceptable for men to work in fields that were technically designated for women. Teachers, stay-at-home-parenthood, and yes, even nurses are now seeing more and more men entering the field. But with the freedom to choose whatever roles suit them the most, men are facing a lot of challenges, especially in the role of caregiving. Here are a few of the biggest challenges men face in nursing.

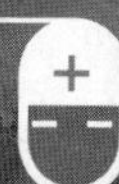

Prejudice in the workplace

In a female-dominated field like nursing, most everything is directed to women. From emails to all the nurses addressed to "ladies" to signage portraying only female nurses, men are often overlooked at work. While none of this is life-threatening, of course, it can still affect male nurses in negative ways. If they see themselves as being treated poorly or forgotten, they might quickly lose motivation to keep doing their job well.

They're seen as untrustworthy

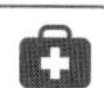

Without a doubt, male nurses receive more negative responses for doing their job than female nurses do. Men in caregiver roles are often seen as having ulterior motives based on some sense of perversion. For some reason, it is still unfathomable to many people that a "big strong man" may want to enter a nurturing profession, and they may see him as a wolf in sheep's clothing. Female patients especially find it difficult to trust male nurses. With many women having had negative experiences with men over the course of their lifetimes, it can be a challenge to allow a man, even in a professional setting, to touch them, treat them, or go over personal health details with them. Likewise, male patients often balk at being treated by another man, especially where physical touching may be involved.

They're not "supposed" to be compassionate

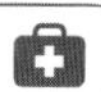

Compassion and empathy are requirements for a great nurse. They are traits that well-rounded, open people possess outside of nursing, too. The problem is that they are seen as feminine traits. From "boys don't cry" to "man up", men are taught from a young age that feelings shouldn't be had or revealed. This does a big disservice to many men who do embody that compassionate nature that is so sought after in the nursing world.

Because so many people hold that mentality, it's difficult for many male nurses to do their work properly. Being constantly looked down on for being a man in a "woman's" role can hurt the ego and impede progress on the part of the nurse. Not to mention, many patients may prefer female nurses instead of male ones because they are perceived to be more compassionate. Thus, many male nurses can lose rapport with patients who might see them as less empathetic.

While we know that this isn't true, men are still facing this myth each day, even though compassion and empathy are not feminine traits, but human ones.

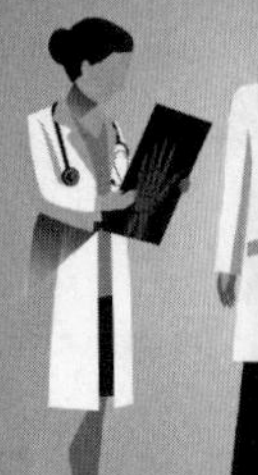

Male nurses are unwelcome in certain specialties 

There are different specialties where men are even less welcome than in others. Labor and delivery, gynecology, even pediatrics are certain departments where most patients may be more comfortable with female nurses. This is most likely because most patients, or parents bringing child patients to the facility, are female. And as we pointed out before, many female patients simply feel less at ease with male nurses.

Especially in gynecology and labor/delivery, where there is often intimate care involved, women may assume that a male nurse is simply in that department for some kind of perverted motive. Many female patients assume that a male nurse cannot provide this type of necessary care without the situation becoming sexual in nature. With female nurses, there is not so much concern.

Male nurses "should" be doctors 

Finally, many male nurses are looked down on because they are nurses and not doctors. For some reason, despite there being both female and male doctors and nurses, it is often presumed that a woman is satisfied with being "just" a nurse, while men should aim for a "higher" goal of being a doctor.

As a nurse you know that becoming a nurse is not a step to becoming a doctor, so there's no reason to assume any nurses simply stopped progressing. Becoming a nurse is a worthy goal in and of itself, for both men and women, and has nothing to do with becoming a doctor. Unfortunately, many men in nursing experience condescension for not having higher goals or motivation to be a doctor.

Final thoughts 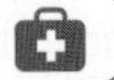

Clearly, being a male nurse is a challenging position. They are often looked down upon by others, discriminated against, and judged. However, the truth is also apparent: there is a growing need for men in nursing. With growing needs for representation in the workplace, you should consider becoming a male nurse if you have a knack for nurturing and want to help people in an important way.

Source: Nursetogether. 2020. Men in nursing: The challenges in caregiving. Retrieved October 26, 2020, from Nursetogether website.

Unit 3 Nursing

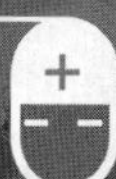

I. Match the words with their definitions according to Passage 1.

____ 1. relic	(a) behaviour that most people think is not normal or acceptable, especially when it is connected with sex
____ 2. ulterior	(b) be reluctant to tackle sth. because it is difficult, dangerous, unpleasant, etc.
____ 3. perversion	(c) sth. that belonged to earlier period but has survived into the present
____ 4. unfathomable	(d) having a variety of experiences and abilities and a fully developed personality
____ 5. empathy	(e) too strange or difficult to be understood
____ 6. balk	(f) to express or represent an idea or a quality
____ 7. well-rounded	(g) (formal) to delay or stop the progress of sth.
____ 8. embody	(h) (of a reason for doing sth.) that sb. keeps hidden and does not admit
____ 9. impede	(i) the ability to understand another person's feelings, experience, etc.
____ 10. rapport	(j) a friendly relationship in which people understand each other very well

II. Read Passage 1 and answer the following questions.

1. What does the author imply by saying "we no longer need to rely on biological relics"?

____

2. Why is nursing not a male-dominated field?

____

3. What does the phrase "a wolf in a sheep's clothing" mean in Paragraph 4?

____

4. Why are male nurses considered to be uncompassionate and unsympathetic?

____

5. What will be the trend for the future nursing staff?

____

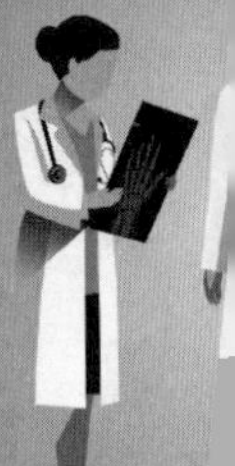

Passage 2 2020: Unleashing the Full Potential of Nursing

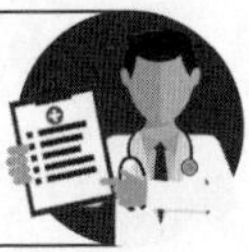

In December, the UK's nursing profession will celebrate the centenary of the Nurses Registration Act 1919, which set training and education standards for nursing and introduced regulation of the profession. This milestone nicely segues into 2020, designated by WHO as the first ever international year of the nurse and midwife. 2020 was chosen to honour the 200th anniversary of the birth of Florence Nightingale—nursing's most iconic figure—who cared for soldiers during the Crimean War and established nursing as a respectable profession for women. There is hope now that nurses and midwives, who are the backbone of primary health-care systems worldwide, will at last receive the recognition, support, and development they deserve.

The value of nursing is almost inestimable. Nurses and midwives make up nearly half of the global health workforce, with around 20 million nurses and 2 million midwives worldwide. Working in a wide variety of roles and in many different contexts, nurses are often the first and only health professionals people see for their health-care needs. Nursing is essential to meeting the challenges posed by demographic changes and rising health-care demands. To achieve the Sustainable Development Goals and respond to humanitarian crises and climate change, among other challenges, whole-of-life care requires a more holistic approach, which nurses are well positioned to deliver. Also, nurses and midwives have a central role in universal health coverage (UHC). Nurse-led clinics could allow rapid and cost-effective expansion of services for non-communicable diseases, advanced nurse practitioners and nurse specialists could strengthen primary care, and nurses could be at the forefront of public health promotion and prevention campaigns and interventions.

Yet, for all its importance, nursing remains underappreciated. Perhaps the biggest barrier that continues to stifle the profession concerns gender and stereotypes. Most nurses are women, and nursing is still viewed by many as women's work and as a soft science, rather than as the highly skilled profession it really is. This perception can also deter men from entering the field. Discrimination exists in the form of low pay and poor working conditions; female nurses are also often overlooked for promotion because of their child-bearing status. Nursing needs to be inclusive of both men and women and represent ethnic minorities, especially in senior management.

Discussions and research around UHC have centred on design and financing; far less attention has been paid to the health-care workforce. More evidence on the role of nurses in primary care is sorely needed. For example, provision of care by lung nurse specialists has been shown to improve clinical outcomes for patients with lung cancer. Such findings can drive policy makers to strengthen investment in nursing, and cost analyses can help make an economic case for supporting the profession.

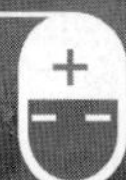

Further initiatives are aiming to address nursing gaps. The aptly named Nightingale Challenge will call on every large employer of nurses to provide leadership and development training for young nurses and midwives (aged 35 years and younger) in 2020, so they can have an even more influential role in global health. These nurses will lobby their respective parliaments on important issues of nursing in an event in October, 2020. Also welcome is the Queen's Nursing Institute's new International Community Nursing Observatory, which will use data-driven analysis to understand community nursing and inform health-care service planning and delivery.

Nursing Now—launched in 2018 by Lord Nigel Crisp and Elizabeth Iro to improve health globally by raising the status of nurses and midwives—has been instrumental in advancing the nursing agenda. On World Health Day (April 7, 2020), in collaboration with Nursing Now and the International Council of Nurses, WHO will publish its first-ever State of the World's Nursing Report. The report should provide analysis of the nursing workforce in member states and examples of best practice, which hopefully will lead to a global nursing strategy. The year of the nurse will continue into 2021 with the publication of the State of the World's Midwifery Report.

These initiatives are laudable, but we are a long way from realising the full value of nursing. If you enhance nursing, you enhance health care. Governments and health systems worldwide should recognise the true potential of nurses. The next 2 years will provide an opportunity to showcase the evidence and impact of what nurses and midwives do and to ensure they are enabled, resourced, and supported to meet the world's health needs.

Source: *The Lancet* Editorial Team. 2019, November 23. 2020: Unleashing the full potential of nursing. *The Lancet*.

I. Match the words with their definitions according to Passage 2.

____ 1. segue	ⓐ to provide sth. with the money or equipment that is needed
____ 2. backbone	ⓑ to move smoothly and unhesitatingly from one state, condition, situation, or element to another
____ 3. stifle	ⓒ a fixed idea or image that many people have of a particular type of person or thing, but which is often not true in reality
____ 4. stereotype	ⓓ to try to influence public officials on behalf of or against (proposed legislation, for example)
____ 5. sorely	ⓔ to prevent sth. from happening
____ 6. aptly	ⓕ very much
____ 7. lobby	ⓖ the most important part of a system, an organization, etc. that

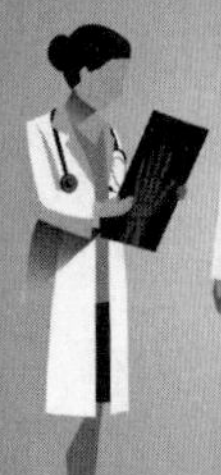

	gives it support and strength
____ 8. laudable	h to exhibit or display
____ 9. showcase	i named, described etc. in a way that seems very suitable
____ 10. resource	j (formal) deserving to be praised or admired, even if not really successful

II. Read Passage 2 and answer the following questions.

1. What is the writing background of the passage?

____

2. Why are nurses and midwives important according to the passage?

____

3. What is the current status for nursing?

____

4. What could be the stereotypes of nurses?

____

5. What is the future trend of nurses and midwives according to the passage?

____

Passage 3 If Nurses Nurse, Why Don't Doctors Doctor?

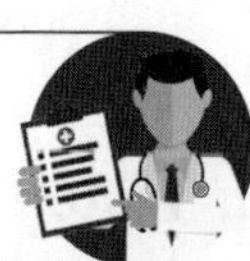

It is a curious feature of the English language that permits nurses to engage in nursing but is disinclined to allow doctors to engage in doctoring—for doctoring carries connotations of nefariousness with which doctors are not normally, and nor would they wish to be, associated. Assuming no historical or present cunning plan to keep nurses in line and while wishing to avoid accusations of paranoia, this limiting feature of the designation "nurse" extends beyond mere curiosity into the realm of perceptions, stereotypes, and myths regarding the description of the roles of nurses and doctors. Perhaps this language feature is no accident after all?

Nurses are nurses, right? Doctors can be physicians, surgeons, pediatricians, geriatricians, pathologists, radiologists, family (or general) practitioners, and so on while nurses can be, well, nurses. In those countries that have a strong association with the British medical system, doctors who are surgeons can be conferred with the title Mr. or Mrs. or Miss or Ms. on obtaining specified qualifications, reflecting a level of expertise beyond that of regular surgical doctors—a badge of honour and status apparently even though each of those titles of Mr. or Mrs. or Miss or Ms. is readily available to non-doctors. Confusingly, at least to outsiders, doctors need not be medical doctors at all; doctors can be doctors of philosophy by virtue of doctoral study leading to the award of a doctorate. And then there are clinical doctorates, professional doctorates, and various forms of course-based doctorates to add to the general confusion of what it means to hold the title doctor. And there are, of course, nurses with doctorates, which make them both nurses and doctors. In some countries, notably North America, the term physician is commonly used to describe medical practitioners and more generally is used sometimes, but not always, to distinguish between the practice of medicine (physicians) and the practice of surgery (surgeons). Thus, doctors may or may not be medical doctors; medical doctors may be physicians or surgeons; and physicians may be surgeons. Further, doctors may be house officers, senior house officers, registrars, interns, residents, consultants, and so on. In North America, doctors might be dentists. And all the while nurses are, well, nurses.

Admittedly, there are some titles that nurses can aspire to—matron and sister spring to mind but by and large, most nurses are known as nurses. Titles available to nurses rarely stray from the root word nurse. The title registered nurse reflects a specified level of qualification and is legally protected in many countries. Staff nurse is commonly used as a job title for a registered nurse, and a staff nurse working in a surgical unit might consider himself or herself to have a specialty although that specialty is not reflected in any generally accepted nursing title. But in some countries, staff nurse might merely mean a nurse who is on the staff of an organization as opposed to a nurse who is freelance. There are some titles for nurses with specialist expertise such as nurse practitioner, advanced practitioner, and consultant nurse but notice how few of these titles do not feature the word nurse or some derivative of that word.

In contrast, there are a number of meanings of the word doctor. One meaning of the verb to doctor implies corruption. To say that a document has been doctored would be to say that that document has been altered so as to mislead the reader; often for the purpose of practising deceit in such a way as to obscure unfavourable outcomes. An accountant accused of doctoring the books would be understood as attempting to show a healthy bank balance where one did not exist for the purpose of personal financial gain. A researcher accused of doctoring data would be understood as seeking to fabricate results to fit a hypothesis or to maintain a reputation. Similarly, a nurse accused of doctoring patient records would be understood as attempting to falsify events so as to cover up an error or an omission. There are a number of meanings of the word nurse but as a verb, to nurse does not lend itself to the kind of negative connotations that can be associated with the verb to doctor.

Thus, to say that nurses nurse is not open to the kind of negative interpretation available when saying that doctors doctor and this may go some way to explaining why common parlance permits

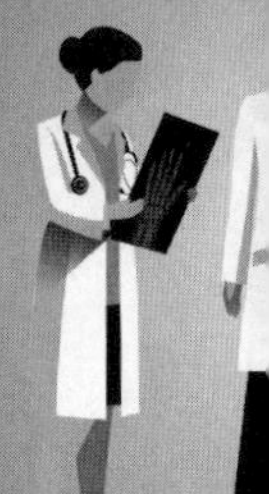

doctors more words for practice than allowed to nurses. Doctors practise medicine whereas nurses practise nursing. Doctors do not, on the whole, practise doctoring. The negative connotations attached to the idea of doctoring are not consistent with the professed values and intentions of doctors despite the attempt by Mol to rehabilitate the term doctoring to describe work for health based on a logic of care rather than a logic of choice.

There is, however, no reason for nurses to become smug with the recognition that the word nurse remains relatively immune from the negative associations to which the word doctor can be subjected for, as outlined above, this same feature of language restricts descriptions of nursing in ways that doctors can transcend with ease—albeit with an associated danger of confusion and imprecision. Thus, linguistically at least, it is truer to say a nurse is a nurse than it is to say a doctor is a doctor. Whether or not this linguistic limitation has been translated into a clinical constraint for nurses will likely forever remain an open question.

Source: Sellman, D. 2015. If nurses nurse, why don't doctors doctor?. *Nursing Philosophy, 16:* 75-76.

I. Match the words with their definitions according to Passage 3.

____ 1. cunning	ⓐ to give sb. a particular honour or right
____ 2. paranoia	ⓑ an advanced student of medicine, whose training is nearly finished and who is working in a hospital to get further practical experience
____ 3. confer	ⓒ mental illness in which a person is obsessed by mistaken beliefs, especially that he is being badly treated by others or that he is somebody very important
____ 4. outsider	ⓓ earning money by selling your work or services to several different organizations rather than being employed by one particular organization
____ 5. expertise	ⓔ a person who is not part of a particular organization or profession
____ 6. smug	ⓕ a doctor working in a hospital in the US who is receiving special advanced training
____ 7. intern	ⓖ to change a written record or information so that it is no longer true
____ 8. resident	ⓗ expert knowledge or skill in a particular subject, activity or job

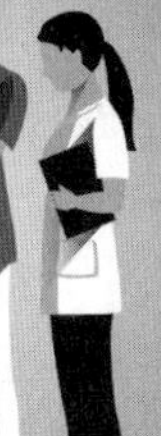

_____ 9. falsify — ❶ (disapproving) able to get what you want in a clever way, especially by tricking or deceiving sb.

_____ 10. freelance — ❶ (disapproving) looking or feeling too pleased about sth. you have done or achieved

II. Read Passage 3 and answer the following questions.

1. Why don't doctors doctor?

____

2. Why do nurses nurse?

____

3. What could be the titles of nurses according to the passage?

____

4. List the meanings of "doctor" mentioned in the passage.

____

5. Is it a good thing for the word "nurse" to remain relatively immune from the negative associations according to the passage? And why?

____

III. Read the three passages comprehensively and answer the following questions.

1. What is the common theme of the three passages?

____

2. What is the main writing skill of Passage 3?

____

3. In your opinion, what is the current status of nursing in China?

____

4. Write a short passage of about 100 words to synthesize the information of the three passages.

____

____

____

____

____

____

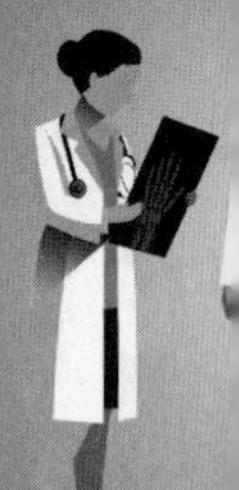

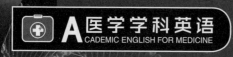

Part C | Integrated Exercises

I. Read the words below, and pay attention to the pronunciation. Use the scale below (1, 2, 3) to give yourself a score for each word. Try to consult your dictionary for the words with score 1.

❶ I don't understand this word.

❷ I understand this word when I see it or hear it, but I don't know how to use it.

❸ I know this word and can use it in my own speaking and writing.

Academic words

□ aptly	□ aspire	□ backbone	□ compassionate
□ condescension	□ confer	□ confusingly	□ connotation
□ cunning	□ demographic	□ derivative	□ deserve
□ deter	□ disincline	□ doctorate	□ embody
□ empathy	□ evolutionarily	□ expertise	□ fabricate
□ falsify	□ forefront	□ freelance	□ humanitarian
□ iconic	□ impede	□ imprecision	□ inestimable
□ laudable	□ launch	□ linguistically	□ lobby
□ mislead	□ nefariousness	□ notably	□ obscure
□ observatory	□ outsider	□ paranoia	□ parlance
□ perception	□ perversion	□ portray	□ profess
□ rapport	□ rehabilitate	□ relics	□ reveal
□ segue	□ showcase	□ smug	□ sorely
□ stereotype	□ stifle	□ transcend	□ ulterior
□ unfathomable	□ unleash	□ untrustworthy	□ well-rounded

Discipline-specific words

□ caregiver	□ child-bearing	□ consultant	□ delivery
□ dentist	□ geriatrician	□ gynecology	□ immune
□ intern	□ irradiation	□ labor	□ matron

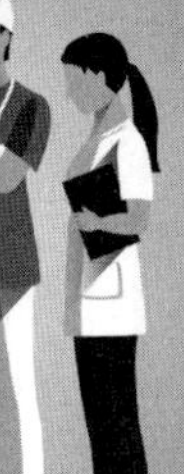

□ mentality	□ midwife	□ midwifery	□ non-communicable
□ nurse	□ pathologist	□ pediatrician	□ pediatrics
□ physician	□ practitioner	□ radiologist	□ registrar
□ resident	□ surgeon	□ surgical	

II. Match each word in the box with the group of words that regularly occur in academic writing.

fabricate	portray	mislead	transcend	pose
launch	deserve	unleash	rehabilitate	reveal

1. ____________ an excuse / evidence / a story
2. ____________ the mystery / the identity / the truth
3. ____________ a situation / a role / a character
4. ____________ reputation / an image / an infrastructure
5. ____________ the public / consumers / readers
6. ____________ boundary / time / limitation
7. ____________ potential / power / energy
8. ____________ attention / respect / recognition
9. ____________ a threat / a problem / a challenge
10. ____________ a business / a satellite / an attack

III. Study the members of the word families in the table below. Try to work out the meaning in each case according to its prefix or suffix.

The members of a word family	Chinese definitions
doctor, doctoral, doctorate	博士、博士的、博士学位
surgeon, surgical, surgery	
pediatric, pediatrics, pediatrician	
note, notable, notably	
precise, precision, imprecision	

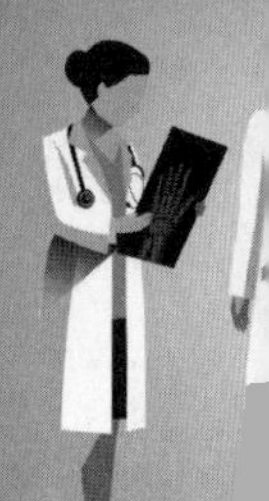

linguistic, linguistics, linguistically	
derive, derivative, derivation	
dental, dentist, dentistry	
pathology, pathologist, pathological	
demography, demographic, demographer	
register, registration, registrar	
promote, promotion, promotional	
humanity, humanitarian, humanitarianism	
perceive, perception, perceptional	
estimate, estimable, inestimable	
observe, observation, observatory	
evolve, evolution, evolutionary, evolutionarily	
motivate, motivation, motivational	
condescend, condescending, condescension	
gynecology, gynecological, gynecologist	

IV. Complete each sentence below with a word from the table above.

1. Lasers are used in a variety of situations in medicine and ________. (surgeon)
2. It can be useful in treating pain and discomfort throughout the body, most ________ in cases of chronic headaches. (note)
3. The robotic systems put a surgeon's hands at the control of a robot with multiple arms and unparalleled ________. (precise)
4. Bad breath is usually caused by a problem in the mouth, so you need to visit your ________ for diagnosis. (dental)
5. There were no significant ________ differences between the screened and unscreened patients. (demography)
6. Two nurses, one consultant and one ________ reviewed patients in the trial. (register)
7. It joined a convey of 23 ambulances and 9 lorries packed with ________ aid. (humanity)

8. ________ speaking, a gene is the particle of inheritance. (evolution)
9. The hypothalamus is one of the most important parts of the brain, involved in many kinds of ________, among other functions. (motivate)
10. A doctor will carry out a pelvic examination and may then arrange further investigations or a referral to a ________. (gynecology)

V. Choose the word in each list that is not a synonym for the underlined word.

1. <u>iconic</u>
   A. symbolic　　B. representative　　C. emblematic　　D. unrecognizable
2. <u>untrustworthy</u>
   A. unreliable　　B. faithful　　C. treacherous　　D. undependable
3. <u>aspire</u>
   A. despise　　B. desire　　C. yearn　　D. strive
4. <u>compassionate</u>
   A. benevolent　　B. merciless　　C. sympathetic　　D. kind
5. <u>confusingly</u>
   A. bewilderedly　　B. puzzlingly　　C. bafflingly　　D. clearly
6. <u>obscure</u>
   A. demonstrate　　B. conceal　　C. hide　　D. veil
7. <u>disincline</u>
   A. indispose　　B. repel　　C. incentivize　　D. deter
8. <u>specified</u>
   A. assigned　　B. designated　　C. appointed　　D. general
9. <u>alter</u>
   A. change　　B. remain　　C. modify　　D. transform
10. <u>restrict</u>
   A. restrain　　B. confine　　C. extend　　D. limit

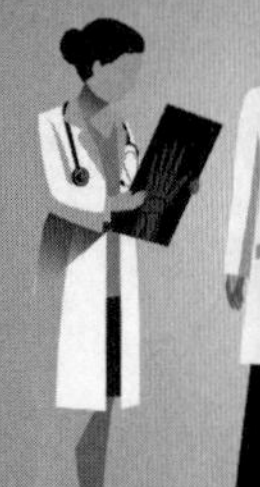

VI. Read the following expressions and sentence patterns aloud and analyze the formality of the structures used.

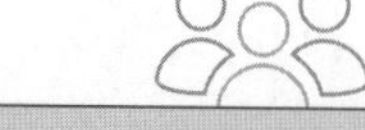

Target sentence patterns

1. **Assuming** no historical or present cunning plan to **keep** nurses **in line** and while wishing to avoid accusations of paranoia, this limiting feature of the designation "nurse" **extends beyond** mere curiosity **into** the realm of perceptions, stereotypes, and myths regarding the description of the roles of nurses and doctors.
2. Doctors can be doctors of philosophy **by virtue of** doctoral study leading to the award of a doctorate.
3. Admittedly, there are some titles that nurses can **aspire to**—matron and sister **spring to mind** but **by and large**, most nurses are known as nurses.
4. But in some countries, staff nurse might merely mean a nurse who is on the staff of an organization **as opposed to** a nurse who is freelance.
5. There are a number of meanings of the word nurse but as a verb, to nurse does not **lend itself to** the kind of negative connotations that can **be associated with** the verb to doctor.
6. Doctors practise medicine **whereas** nurses practise nursing. Doctors do not, **on the whole**, practise doctoring.
7. The negative connotations **attached to** the idea of doctoring **are** not **consistent with** the professed values and intentions of doctors **despite** the attempt by Mol to rehabilitate the term doctoring to describe work for health **based on** a logic of care **rather than** a logic of choice.
8. Working in **a wide variety of** roles and in many different contexts, nurses are often the first and only health professionals people see for their health-care needs.
9. To **achieve** the Sustainable Development **Goals** and **respond to** humanitarian crises and climate change, among other challenges, whole-of-life care requires a more holistic approach, which nurses **are well positioned to** deliver.
10. Nurse-led clinics could allow rapid and cost-effective expansion of services for non-communicable diseases, advanced nurse practitioners and nurse specialists could strengthen primary care, and nurses could **be at the forefront of** public health promotion and prevention campaigns and interventions.
11. This perception can also **deter** men **from** entering the field.
12. Discussions and research around UHC **have centred on** design and financing; **far less**

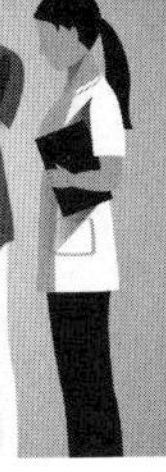

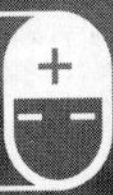

attention has been paid to the health-care workforce.

13. The year of the nurse will continue into 2021 **with the publication of** the State of the World's Midwifery Report.
14. On World Health Day (April 7, 2020), **in collaboration with** Nursing Now and the International Council of Nurses, WHO will publish its first-ever State of the World's Nursing Report.
15. Instead, as an advanced species, we **have the luxury of making our** own proper **decisions** that are best for us, our lives, and the people we care about, **regardless of** what our DNA might say.
16. **It hasn't been until** recent years **that** it's become more acceptable for men to work in fields that **were** technically **designated for** women.
17. **Without a doubt**, male nurses receive more negative responses for doing their job than female nurses do.
18. With many women having had negative experiences with men over the course of their lifetimes, it can be a challenge to allow a man, even in a professional setting, to touch them, treat them, or **go over** personal health details with them.
19. Likewise, male patients often **balk at** being treated by another man, especially where physical touching may be involved.
20. This **does a big disservice to** many men who do embody that compassionate nature that **is so sought after** in the nursing world.
21. **Being** constantly **looked down on** for being a man in a "woman's" role can hurt the ego and impede progress on the part of the nurse.
22. Thus, many male nurses can **lose rapport with** patients who might see them as less empathetic.
23. And **as** we **pointed out** before, many female patients simply **feel less at ease with** male nurses.
24. For some reason, **despite** there being both female and male doctors and nurses, it is often presumed that a woman **is satisfied with** being "just" a nurse, while men should **aim for** a "higher" goal of being a doctor.
25. However, the truth is also apparent: **there is a growing need for** men in nursing. With growing needs for representation in the workplace, you should consider becoming a male nurse if you **have a knack for** nurturing and want to help people in an important way.

VII. For each of the sentences below, write a new sentence as similar as possible in meaning to the original one, but as formal as possible in style.

1. If there is no increase in food intake, you can lose ten pounds in a year's time.

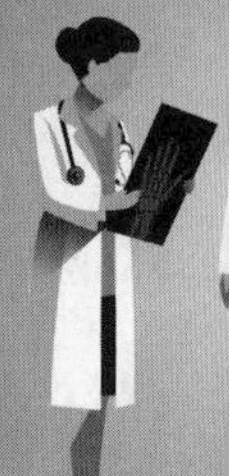

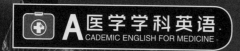

2. He finally survived this infectious disease with his will power.

3. When you think of the fertility problem, what you firstly think of may be Africa.

4. Generally speaking, this operation might have had more negative than positive effects.

5. He was the first scientist to identify embryonic stem cells, which can be adapted for different kinds of medical purposes.

6. It evokes what it feels like to be the most advanced stage in the development of modern biomedicine and to bring new knowledge and technologies into the clinic.

7. Even biology undergraduates may reject animal experiments.

8. We harm ourselves greatly when we condemn the healthy desires behind temptation.

9. Headed out the door with your health concerns addressed, you're much more likely to be less worried than during the anticipation of first seeing the doctor.

10. IgE antibodies are closely connected to certain cells, called mast cells, in tissue throughout the body.

VIII. Translate the following sentences by using the following words and phrases. Make sure that your English sentences are different from the Chinese versions in terms of structures or orders, but as formal as possible. Then compare yours with your partner's according to the criteria: Whose version is more different and more formal?

1. 拥有健康生活的一个最好方式是增加每天的行走时间。(keep in line)

   ____

2. 总的来说，怀孕期间的饮食注意事项和其他时期是一致的。(by and large)

   ____

3. 无烟烟草的使用似乎也与血压升高相关。(be associated with)

   ____

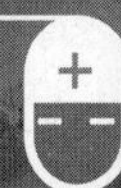

4. 因为很多问题尚未解决，病毒可能还会通过医疗途径传播到其他物种中。 (lend itself to)

____

5. 吸烟会导致癌症、心脏病和许多其他疾病，因此，人们不应因为担心适当的增重而放弃戒烟。(deter from)

____

6. 世界卫生组织已经与几个会员国开展合作，发送用于外科手术和创伤干预的医疗用品。(in collaboration with)

____

7. 随着本书的出版，心理治疗终于成为心理健康实践的主流。(with the publication of)

____

8. 心肌细胞是再生医疗中最紧缺的细胞之一。(be sought after)

____

9. 护士与患者之间的关系变得不再融洽，技术是否要对此负责？ (lose rapport with)

____

10. 针灸学校的需求日益增长。(There is a growing need for)

____

Part D Academic Skills

Academic Listening Skill

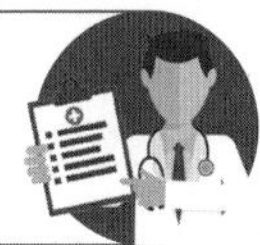

Finding the Sequence of Events in a Narrative

When you listen to a narrative, it is important to follow the sequence of events so that you do not lose the track of an event. An effective way is to listen for specific periods of time, dates, years or some other time expressions such as “firstly”, “a few years later”, “after a while”, “then”, and “in the end”. Usually, we can follow the sequence of events in a narrative, if we put together the information that follows such time expressions.

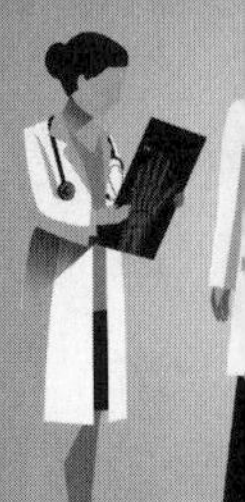

Listening 1

Word bank

1. bandage	a long, narrow piece of cloth that is tied around an injury or a part of someone's body that has been hurt
2. lamp	a device for giving light, especially one that has a covering or is contained within sth.
3. heroin	a woman who is admired for having done sth. very brave or having achieved sth. great
4. amazing	very good
5. merit	the quality of being good and deserving praise

I. Listen to the passage and complete the chart below.

Florence Nightingale's Life Story	
Time	**Event**
In ________	Nightingale's parents went to ________ after they got married.
In ________	Nightingale went to Germany and learned all about ________.
In ________	Nightingale and ________ nurses went to help at the Crimean War.
At night at the hospitals	Nightingale walked around to talk to the ________ and helped them to ________ to their families.
When she ________ to England	People called her a ________ because of her amazing work in the Crimean War.
After the war	Nightingale continued to work hard in ________ to ________.

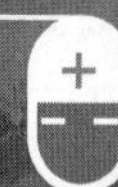

II. Listen to the passage and choose the right answer to each of the questions.

❶ **What does the passage mainly talk about?**

A Why Queen Victoria wrote Florence Nightingale a letter.

B Why Florence Nightingale's parents worried about her decision of becoming a nurse.

C How Florence Nightingale took care of the wounded British soldiers at the Crimean War.

D What achievements of Florence Nightingale got and her contributions to nursing in the 19th century.

❷ **Which of the following options is NOT correct?**

A Florence Nightingale brought wounded soldiers fresh food.

B Due to Nightingale's hard work, fewer Britain soldiers died at the Crimean War.

C Nightingale continued to dedicate to nursing work when the Crimean War finished.

D Nightingale aspired to be a nurse and help people because she did not want to be married.

Listening 2

Word bank

1. specialty	a pursuit, area of study or skill to which someone has devoted much time and effort and in which they are expert
2. supervise	to observe and direct the execution of (a task, project, or activity)
3. doctoral	relating to or designed to achieve a doctorate
4. prescribe	to advise and authorize the use of (a medicine or treatment) for someone, especially in writing
5. LPN	abbr. Licensed Practical Nurse
6. RN	abbr. Registered Nurse
7. APN	abbr. Advanced Practice Nurse

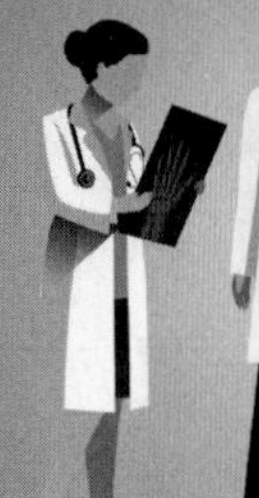

I. Listen to the passage and choose the right answer to each of the questions.

❶ Which of the following statements is NOT the nurses' responsibility?

Ⓐ Nurses are responsible for the treatment, care and safety of patients.
Ⓑ Nurses are responsible for maintenance of health and education for the patient.
Ⓒ Nurses provide direct care and monitor symptoms, response, and progress in patient care.
Ⓓ Nurses are responsible for the doctors and under the supervision of the doctors.

❷ Which of the following is the best tile of the passage?

Ⓐ Types of Nurse
Ⓑ Responsibilities of Nurse
Ⓒ Hospital Nurse
Ⓓ The Art of Nursing

II. Listen carefully and then write down the degrees, responsibilities or specialties of LPN, RN and APN.

Type	Degree	Responsibility / Specialties
LPN	usually ________ of training	1. They perform simple and some complex ________ ________. 2. The work ________ to provide patient care.
RN	has a ________ degree in ________	1. They ________, ________ and ________ about proper patient care. 2. They are responsible for ________.
APN	has a ________ or ________ degree	1. They provide direct care, diagnose disease, ________ ________, ________ and educate patients and other health care professionals. 2. There are many ________ for them.

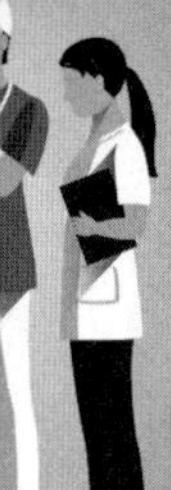

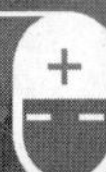

Academic Reading Skill

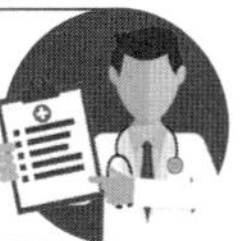

Signal Words

Signal words give hints about what is going to happen in the text. Signal words are keys to comprehension. Highlighting signal words is a useful strategy since it helps readers understand the passage better. Signal words are useful in identifying author's view, understanding the structure and locating key information for questions. In this chapter, we'll mainly focus on transitional signal words. They can be divided into several types: to introduce an additional idea, to compare and contrast, to show concession, to introduce causes and effects, to give examples, to show chronological order, to show order of importance, to show alternatives, to identify or clarify, to reinforce and to conclude.

- Signals that **introduce an additional idea** include but are not limited to: *also, besides, furthermore, in addition, moreover, additionally, and, or, another +noun, an additional + noun*.
- Signals that **compare and contrast** include but are not limited to: *likewise, similarly, equally, however, whereas, while, in contrast, differ from, on the other hand, in the same way, both...and, neither... nor, just as, as...as*.
- Signals that **show concession** aim to show an unexpected result. They include but are not limited to, like *although, however, yet, nevertheless, nonetheless, still, though, despite, in spite of*.
- Signals that **introduce causes and effects** include but are not limited to: *for this reason, for, because, since, as, result from, a result of, an effect of, as a result, consequently, hence, thus, therefore, so, result in, the cause of*.
- Signals that **give examples i**nclude but are not limited to: *for example, for instance, in this case, such as*.
- Signals that **show chronological order** are commonly seen in any writing like: *first, second, first of all, then, before, after, until, previously, since, when, finally,* to name just a few.
- Signals that **show alternatives** include but are not limited to: *alternatively, otherwise, or, if, unless*.
- Signals for the purpose of **identifying and clarifying** include but are not limited to: *that is, in other words, specifically, namely, i.e.*

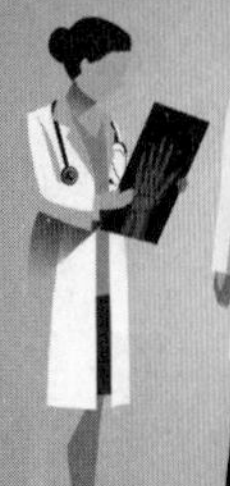

- Signals of **reinforcing** include but are not limited to: *in fact, indeed, of course, and clearly.*
- Signals of **conclusion** include but are not limited to: *all in all, in brief, in conclusion, in short, in summary.*

To summarize, signals differ in their functions. To grasp the structure of a passage and stick author's ideas together, it requires readers to notice signals while reading.

I. Read the following paragraphs and underline the signal words.

❶ Because so many people hold that mentality, it's difficult for many male nurses to do their work properly. Being constantly looked down on for being a man in a "woman's" role can hurt the ego and impede progress on the part of the nurse. Not to mention, many patients may prefer female nurses instead of male ones because they are perceived to be more compassionate. Thus, many male nurses can lose rapport with patients who might see them as less empathetic.

❷ Yet, for all its importance, nursing remains underappreciated. Perhaps the biggest barrier that continues to stifle the profession concerns gender and stereotypes. Most nurses are women, and nursing is still viewed by many as women's work and as a soft science, rather than as the highly skilled profession it really is. This perception can also deter men from entering the field. Discrimination exists in the form of low pay and poor working conditions; female nurses are also often overlooked for promotion because of their child-bearing status. Nursing needs to be inclusive of both men and women and represent ethnic minorities, especially in senior management.

❸ There is, however, no reason for nurses to become smug with the recognition that the word nurse remains relatively immune from the negative associations to which the word doctor can be subjected for, as outlined above, this same feature of language restricts descriptions of nursing in ways that doctors can transcend with ease—albeit with an associated danger of confusion and imprecision. Thus, linguistically at least, it is truer to say a nurse is a nurse than it is to say a doctor is a doctor. Whether or not this linguistic limitation has been translated into a clinical constraint for nurses will likely forever remain an open question.

II. Read the following passage and fill in the blanks where the first letter of each word or phrase has been given.

The report provides up-to-date information on the global nursing workforce, including on the overall shortage of nurses, estimated at almost 6 million—with the vast majority of shortfalls in

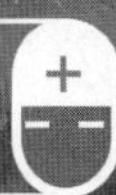

low-income and middle-income countries, where the growth in nurse numbers is scarcely keeping pace with population growth. **B**________ even in some high-income countries the demand for nurses outpaces their supply: in England, in 2019 there were about 40,000 vacancies for nurse roles across health and care settings. **M**________, the need for wealthier countries **s**________ **a**________ the UK and Germany to recruit from abroad can contribute to the workforce shortages in other countries. **A**________ **t**________ the WHO report, the number of nurse graduates worldwide will need to increase by an average of 8% per year to overcome the global shortage by 2030. Across various settings at all levels of the health system, from routine clinic visits to inpatient care, nurses have a central role in caring for people with diabetes. **I**________ **p**________, the IDF emphasizes the key contributions of nurses in ensuring the timely diagnosis of diabetes, in helping to prevent type 2 diabetes by addressing risk factors, and in the provision of self-management education and psychological support for patients.

➢ To find more information about signal words, you may refer to the following sources.

1. Office of Academics and Transformation, Department of English Language Arts. 2020. Transitional signal words. Retrieved August 27, 2020, from Language Arts Reading website.
2. Smith, S. 2020. Transition signals. Retrieved August 27, 2020, from EAPFOUNDATION website.

Academic Writing Skill

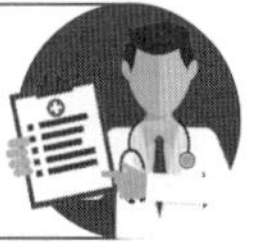

Comparison and Contrast

Writing an essay with comparison and contrast requires you to examine how things are similar (comparison) and to analyze how things differ (contrast). This process usually involves a deep understanding and critical thinking to generate analysis and clarify meaningful connections between two or more subjects (items, ideas, theories, researches, etc.) based on certain criteria. Before writing the essay, you'd better brainstorm and draft a Venn diagram as shown below to list the pros and cons of each subject you are comparing or contrasting.

As many other types of essay, you may need to outline comparison and contrast essay into introduction part (what you will discuss and why your readers should care), body part (provide evidence to support your argument), and conclusion part (summarize the essay and restate the thesis). Sometimes the whole essay will compare and contrast, though sometimes the comparison

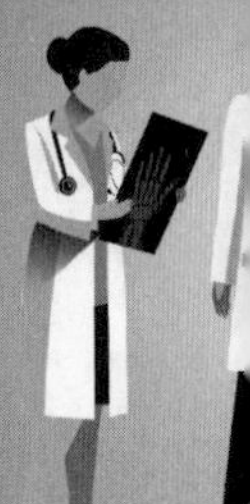

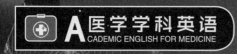

or contrast may be only part of the essay (for example, as a preliminary stage of evaluation). It is also possible, especially for short exam essays (*Coffee vs. Tea: Which One Is Healthier*), that only the similarities or the differences, not both, will be discussed.

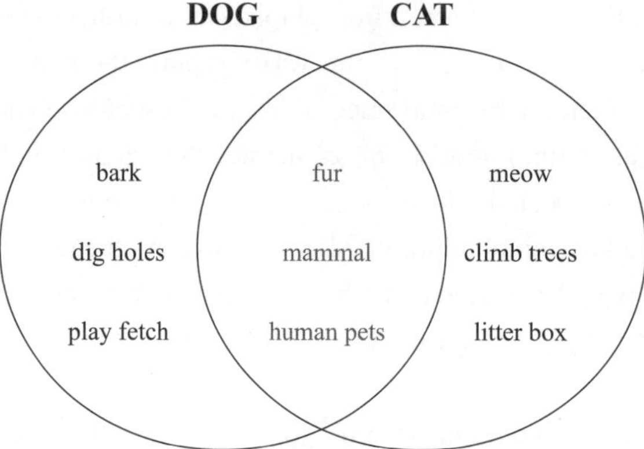

Commonly, there are mainly two ways to structure a comparison and contrast essay:

1) **Block Structure**: deals with all of the points about the first subject being compared or contrasted, and then moves on to list all of the points about the second subject (then the third, and so on, if you're comparing or contrasting more than two subjects).
2) **Point-by-Point Structure:** deals with one point of comparison/contrast between/among subjects at a time, followed by the similarity (or difference) for the other points.

Block Structure
Subject 1–Point 1
Subject 1–Point 2
Subject 1–Point 3…
Subject 2–Point 1
Subject 2–Point 2
Subject 2–Point 3…
…

Point-by-point Structure
Point 1 Subject 1 ➢ Subject 2 ➢ …
Point 2 Subject 1 ➢ Subject 2 ➢ …
Point 3 Subject 1 ➢ Subject 2 ➢ …
…

Both types of structure have their merits. The former one can make your essay smoother and is relatively easier to write, while the latter one makes what you're comparing and contrasting clearer. Choose the structure that can make readers keep track of your argumentation.

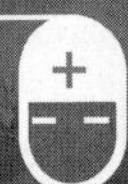

To keep your argumentation cohesive, it is helpful to use signal words and phrases in the table below to indicate similarities or differences and to cue readers the content and organization of your analysis.

Comparison	Contrast
both, like, also, likewise, similarly, similar to, just like, in the same way, to compare (to/with), as... as..., neither... nor..., the same as...	instead, while, however, whereas, but, yet, nevertheless, unlike, conversely, in contrast, on the contrary, not so... as..., different (from), (on the one hand)...on the other hand...

I. Read Passage 3 and decide the following statements are true (T) or false (F).

1. This passage focuses on contrasting doctors and nurses without comparing. (　　)
2. The author uses the linguistic criteria to make a contrast between doctors and nurses. (　　)
3. The author believes that it is merely in the title that doctors are different from nurses. (　　)
4. According to the author, nurse is a word with linguistic limitation and has just one meaning while doctor has many meanings and is more advanced and noble. (　　)

II. Read the paragraph below and do the following exercises.

Although LVNs and RNs work closely together, they have different nursing scope of practices. Both LVNs and RNs provide client care using clinical skills, knowledge, and judgement. However, an RN has more in-depth clinical knowledge and experience, and is able to perform more complex duties in comparison to the LVN. With regard to assessment, it is the first step of the nursing process. After client health information is gathered, the RN will use clinical judgement and thinking to verify, analyze, and interpret the collected health information to form the client's plan of care, develop a care plan, and to address other factors affecting the client. RNs work independently while LVNs work under the supervision of the registered nurse and physician. Although both LVNs and RNs participate in the assessment phase, the RN is responsible for overseeing and supervising the entire nursing process.

❶ This paragraph is ________.

Ⓐ a comparison paragraph　　Ⓑ a contrast paragraph　　Ⓒ both

❷ Fill in the table with the criteria and contents of comparison and contrast between LVNs and RNs.

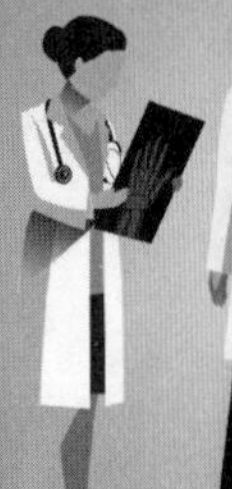

	Criteria	LVNs	RNs
Comparison			
Contrast			

III. Complete the comparison and contrast sentences by choosing from the list of sentences in the table below.

1. Conventional medicine focuses on the factors that cause diseases; every abnormality is seen as an independent clause, separate from the personality of an individual and their environment.

   ____

2. Alternative medicine assumes health is a life-long process; therefore, to sustain a healthy body condition, a person should continually maintain proper nutrition, daily regimen, body care, mind exercises, and so on.

   ____

3. Organic products such as fruits will always be variable sizes and shapes, presenting some form of physical imperfection compared to their non-organic counterparts.

   ____

4. A food product will only be labeled as organic if it is free of any additives that were made artificially, such as preservatives, flavoring, sweeteners, as well as colorings.

   ____

Ⓐ On the other hand, nonorganic foods will always appear to have a relatively similar appearance in accordance with their various types.

Ⓑ Conventional medicine, while also taking these principles into consideration, relies mostly on drugs and surgery.

Ⓒ On the other hand, inorganic foods are those that are grown using artificial chemicals.

Ⓓ Unlike its counterpart, alternative medicine sees a body as an equilibrium of interrelations between a body and its environment; therefore, disease is thought to be caused by an imbalance between them.

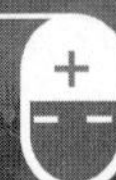

IV. Write a comparison and contrast essay titled "Doctors vs. Nurses". The opening has been given.

Doctors vs. Nurses

In the medical field, doctors and nurses are two groups of people who share an almost indistinguishable goal—to serve the patient to the best of their ability. Yet, although these two professions have a lot in common, there are many differences between them.

…

- **Now check your writing or your peer's writing based on the following checklist.**

Item	Yes or No
The essay is a comparison and contrast essay.	
The essay has a clear thesis statement.	
An appropriate structure is used, either block or point-by-point.	
Signal words and phrases for comparison and contrast are used accurately.	
The criteria for comparison/contrast are clear.	

➢ To find more information about how to write an essay with comparison and contrast, you may refer to the following sources.

1. Fleming, G. 2020. Venn Diagrams to plan essays and more. Retrieved August 26, 2020, from ThoughtCo website.
2. Morgan, M. 2023. How to write a compare and contrast essay. Retrieved January 29, 2023, from Wikihow website.

Unit 4

Mental Health

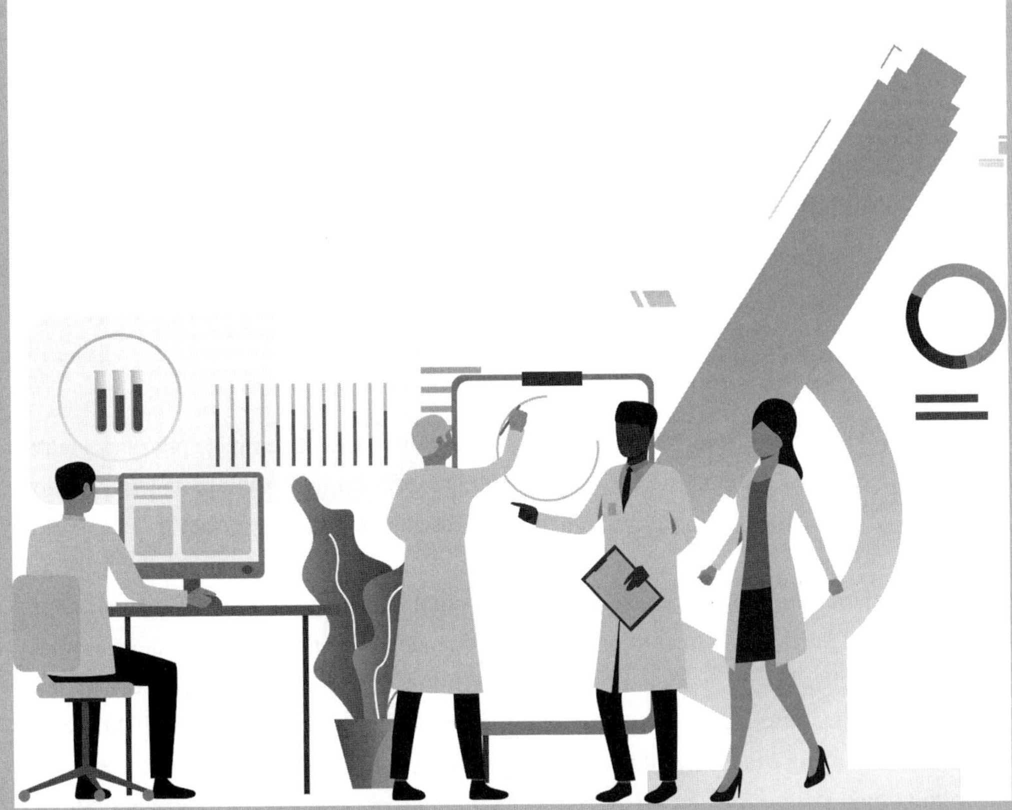

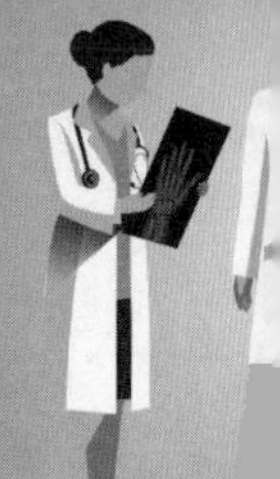

Part A | Information Searching and Delivering

I. Surf on the Internet and find information about the following topics before class.

1. major depression
2. attention deficit hyperactivity disorder (ADHD)
3. schizophrenia
4. post-traumatic stress disorder (PTSD)
5. obsessive-compulsive disorder (OCD)

II. Make a presentation based on the information you've searched.

Part B | Text Understanding

Passage 1 Mental Health and Mental Disorders

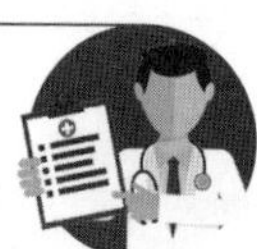

What is mental health and how significant is it? 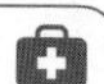

The World Health Organization (WHO) states, "Health is a state of complete physical, mental and social well-being and not merely the absence of disease or infirmity." An important implication of this statement is that mental health is an integral and essential component of health. But what is mental health?

Cultural differences, subjective assessments, and competing professional theories all affect how "mental health" is defined. According to the WHO, mental health includes "subjective well-being, perceived self-efficacy, autonomy, competence, inter-generational dependence, and self-actualization of one's intellectual and emotional potential, among others." The WHO further states that the well-being of an individual is encompassed in the realization of his or her abilities, coping with normal stresses of life, productive work and contribution to their community. It can

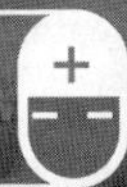

be concluded that mental health is more than just the absence of mental disorders or disabilities. Mental health is a state of well-being in which an individual realizes his or her own individual and collective ability as a human to think, to emote, to handle stresses, to work productively, to interact with each other and to make a contribution to his or her community. The state of being mentally healthy is enviable given the advantages it affords. For example, mentally healthy adults tend to report the fewest health-related limitations of their routine activities, the fewest full or partially missed days of work, and the healthiest social functioning (for example, low helplessness, clear life goals, high resilience, and high levels of intimacy in their lives).

However, unfortunately, it is a sad fact that many people around the world do not experience mental health in these ways. Instead, they suffer from different mental disorders. Mental disorders are more common than cancer, diabetes, or heart disease due to the fact that they can affect anyone regardless of age, gender, social status, religion or race/ethnicity and cultural background. Evidence from the WHO suggests that nearly half of the world's population are affected by mental disorders with an impact on their self-esteem, relationships and ability to function in everyday life. A WHO report estimates the global cost of mental disorders at nearly \$2.5 trillion (two-thirds in indirect costs) in 2010, with a projected increase to over \$6 trillion by 2030.

What is a mental disorder? 

A mental disorder is also called a psychiatric disorder or mental illness. Although debates about how to define a mental disorder have been ongoing for years, the Diagnostic and Statistical Manual of Mental Disorders, 5th Edition (DSM-5) has recently given an updated, if still imperfect, definition of mental disorder as "a syndrome characterized by clinically significant disturbance in an individual's cognition, emotion regulation, or behavior that reflects a dysfunction in the psychological, biological, or developmental processes underlying mental functioning." Put it simply, a mental disorder refers to a behavioral or mental pattern that may cause suffering or a poor ability to function in life since it affects your mood, thinking and behavior.

How to tell whether it is a mental disorder? 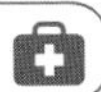

Everyone experiences sadness, anxiety, irritability, and moodiness at times and many people have mental health concerns from time to time. But a mental health concern becomes a mental disorder when ongoing signs and symptoms are severe enough to interfere with the daily activities. Signs and symptoms of a mental disorder can vary in degree of severity, ranging from mild to moderate to severe, but mainly affect the person with it physically, socially and emotionally. A mental disorder can have virtually any physical symptom associated with it, from insomnia, headaches, changes in appetite and energy level, unexplained aches and pains to even paralysis.

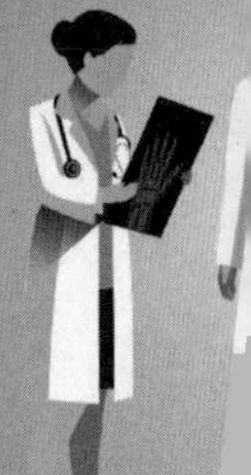

Socially, the person with a mental disorder may suffer from social withdrawal, in which they avoid or have trouble making or keeping friends. Emotionally, the person may have severe mood swings, persistent thoughts or compulsions, and feels sad, helpless, hopeless, or agitated. These emotional problems can even result in the person wanting to commit suicide or hurt others.

If you have been experiencing some of the above signs and symptoms for at least two consecutive weeks, you may be suffering from a mental disorder.

What are the common mental disorders? 

Some of the most common and frequently reported mental disorders include anxiety, depressive, behavioral, and substance abuse disorders.

Anxiety disorders are characterized by excessive worry to the point of interfering with the sufferer's ability to function. Depressive disorders involve feelings of sadness that interfere with the individual's ability to function or, as with adjustment disorder, persist longer than most people experience in reaction to a particular life stressor. Behavioral disorders (like attention deficit hyperactivity disorder [ADHD]) are characterized by problems conforming to the tenets of acceptable behavior. Substance use disorders, like substance abuse and substance dependence, involve the use of a substance that interferes with the social, emotional, physical, educational, or vocational functioning of the person using it.

How to cope with mental disorders? 

The first step towards getting mental disorders addressed is to see a doctor or mental health professional for diagnosis. To diagnose, the doctor will do a mental health assessment, which is a detailed and comprehensive interview, including questions about symptoms and their impact on work and relationships, any previous episodes, drug and alcohol use, medical conditions and family history. It is important to assess the risk of suicide or self-harm.

The second step in the recovery process is to choose the right treatment. Treatment choices for mental disorders will vary from person to person. Even people with the same diagnosis will have different experiences, needs, goals and objectives for treatment. There is no "one size fits all" treatment. Innovations in the range of evidence-based medications, therapy and psychosocial services such as psychiatric rehabilitation, housing, employment and peer supports have made wellness and recovery a reality for people living with mental disorders.

A person cannot be fully healthy in his body unless he is mentally healthy too. Despite the fact that millions of people are not in a position to experience mental health, mental disorders, even the worst case, are treatable. With early diagnosis and treatment, many people can manage their

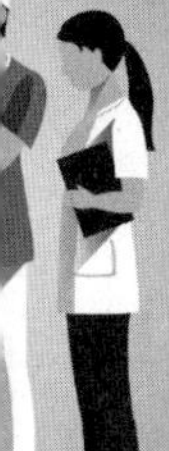

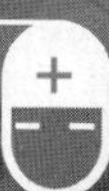

symptoms and even fully recover from their mental disorders.

Sources: 1. Encyclopedia. 2020. Mental health. Retrieved July 25, 2020, from The Free Dictionary website.
2. Nedha. 2011. Difference between mental health and mental illness. Retrieved August 12, 2020, from Difference Between website.
3. NAMI. 2020. Treatments. Retrieved August 15, 2020, from NAMI website.

I. Match the words with their definitions according to Passage 1.

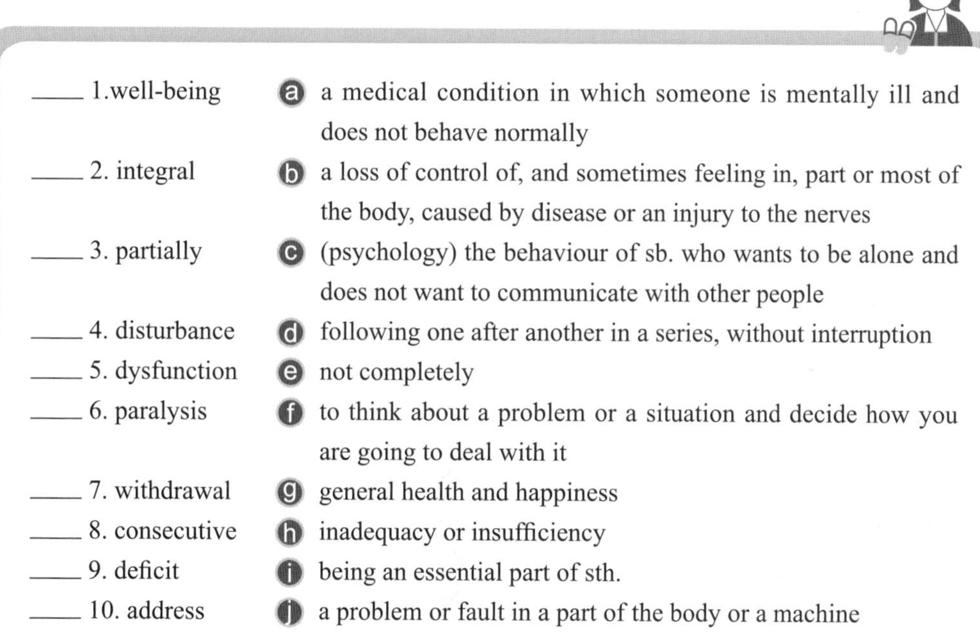

____ 1.well-being	ⓐ a medical condition in which someone is mentally ill and does not behave normally
____ 2. integral	ⓑ a loss of control of, and sometimes feeling in, part or most of the body, caused by disease or an injury to the nerves
____ 3. partially	ⓒ (psychology) the behaviour of sb. who wants to be alone and does not want to communicate with other people
____ 4. disturbance	ⓓ following one after another in a series, without interruption
____ 5. dysfunction	ⓔ not completely
____ 6. paralysis	ⓕ to think about a problem or a situation and decide how you are going to deal with it
____ 7. withdrawal	ⓖ general health and happiness
____ 8. consecutive	ⓗ inadequacy or insufficiency
____ 9. deficit	ⓘ being an essential part of sth.
____ 10. address	ⓙ a problem or fault in a part of the body or a machine

II. Read Passage 1 and answer the following questions.

1. What could be the possible advantages for a mentally healthy adult?

____

2. How can a person tell that he has a mental disorder?

____

3. In what aspects does a mental disorder affect a person and how?

____

4. What does the author mean by saying that there is no "one size fits all" treatment?

____

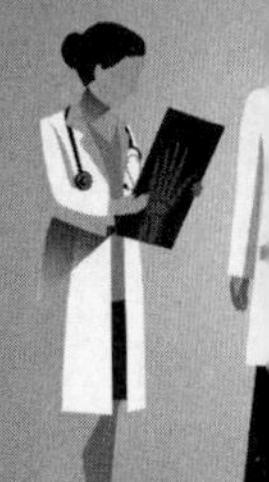

5. What should we do in order to maintain mental health?

____

Passage 2 No Physical Health Without Mental Health: Lessons Unlearned?

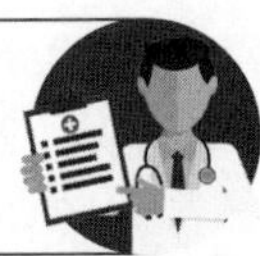

Dr. Brock Chisholm, the first Director-General of the World Health Organization (WHO), was a psychiatrist and shepherded the notion that mental and physical health were intimately linked. He famously stated that "without mental health there can be no true physical health". Half a century later, we have strong evidence elucidating the bidirectional relationship between mental illnesses—specifically depression and anxiety—and physical health outcomes. However, policy continues to lag behind the evidence in this regard, as demonstrated by our global noncommunicable disease response.

Over a decade ago, the World Health Assembly adopted a global strategy for the prevention and control of noncommunicable diseases. At the time, these were limited to the following four illness types: cardiovascular disease, diabetes, respiratory illness and cancers. Such a categorization would set a precedent for the exclusion of mental illnesses from all future WHO discussions on noncommunicable diseases. It is not surprising then, that in the 2008–2013 action plan for the global strategy for the prevention and control of noncommunicable diseases mental illnesses were relegated to a footnote, with the justification that they do not share risk factors with the other four types of illnesses.

We take issue with this viewpoint, as mental illnesses are themselves risk factors that affect the incidence and prognosis of diseases traditionally classified as "noncommunicable". Patients with type II diabetes mellitus, for example, are twice as likely to experience depression as the general population, and those patients with diabetes who are depressed have greater difficulty with self-care. Patients suffering from mental illness are twice as likely to smoke cigarettes as other people, and in patients with chronic obstructive pulmonary disease, mental illness is linked to poorer clinical outcomes. Up to 50% of cancer patients suffer from a mental illness, especially depression and anxiety, and treating symptoms of depression in cancer patients may improve survival time. Similarly, in patients who are depressed, the risk of having a heart attack is more than twice as high as in the general population; further, depression increases the risk of death in patients with cardiac disease. Moreover, treating the symptoms of depression after a heart attack has been shown to lower both mortality and re-hospitalization rates. In light of this evidence, how can we possibly address the burgeoning epidemic of noncommunicable diseases without tackling

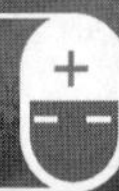

co-morbid mental illnesses?

Mental illnesses were declared a regional priority in Africa during the WHO African Region Ministerial Consultation on Noncommunicable Diseases, held in Brazzaville, Congo, in April 2011. Later that month the WHO's African Member States and India reiterated this priority at the first Global Ministerial Conference on Healthy Lifestyles and Noncommunicable Disease Control, held in Moscow, Russia. As a result, mental illnesses were featured prominently in the preambles of the Moscow Declaration, as well as in the political declaration issued by the United Nations General Assembly at the high-level meeting on noncommunicable diseases held in New York City in September 2011. Despite this progress, however, mental illnesses received no mention at all in the resolution on noncommunicable diseases that WHO's Member States adopted during the 130th session of WHO's Executive Board. Mental illnesses were also omitted from WHO's proposed monitoring framework, indicators and voluntary targets for the prevention and control of noncommunicable diseases, which was released in November 2012.

The 2008–2013 action plan for the global strategy for the prevention and control of noncommunicable diseases will be revised over the coming year, and the WHO's Executive Board and World Health Assembly are preparing their deliberations for 2013. During this critical time, we urge Member States to recognize the importance of co-morbid mental illnesses as amplifiers of the burden of other noncommunicable diseases. To this end, we call on Member States to assess and monitor co-morbid mental illnesses in primary care settings, prioritize the training of professionals in mental health care, and critically incorporate mental health interventions within chronic disease programs as part of a vigorous global response to noncommunicable diseases. We now know that addressing mental illnesses in primary care settings will delay progression, improve survival outcomes, and reduce the health care costs of other noncommunicable diseases. The time has now come to do away with the artificial divisions between mental and physical health, as WHO's first Director-General championed so many decades ago.

Source: Kolappa, K., Henderson, D. C. & Kishore, S. P. 2013. No physical health without mental health: Lessons unlearned? Retrieved August 14, 2020, from PubMed Central website.

I. Match the words with their definitions according to Passage 2.

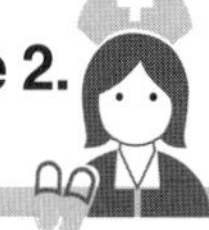

____ 1. shepherd	ⓐ an introduction to a book or a written document
____ 2. relegate	ⓑ to have an important part in sth.
____ 3. prognosis	ⓒ rapidly developing or growing
____ 4. pulmonary	ⓓ the process of carefully considering or discussing sth.

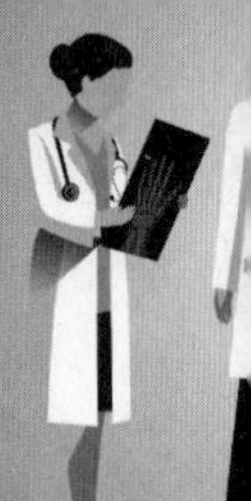

____ 5. burgeoning	e	to guide sb. or a group of people somewhere, making sure they go where you want them to go
____ 6. feature	f	pertaining to the lungs
____ 7. preamble	g	an opinion, based on medical experience, of the likely development of a disease or an illness
____ 8. indicator	h	to fight for or speak in support of a group of people or a belief
____ 9. deliberation	i	to consign to an inferior or obscure place, rank, category, or condition
____ 10. champion	j	a sign that shows you what sth. is like or how a situation is changing

II. Read Passage 2 and answer the following questions.

1. How do you understand the bidirectional relationship between mental illnesses and physical health outcomes?

   ____

2. What is the attitude of the passage toward 2008–2013 action plan?

   ____

3. What does noncommunicable disease refer to according to the passage?

   ____

4. Why should we address the importance of mental illness as equal as that of noncommunicable diseases?

   ____

5. What is the purpose of writing this article?

   ____

Passage 3 Mental Health Care for University Students: A Way Forward?

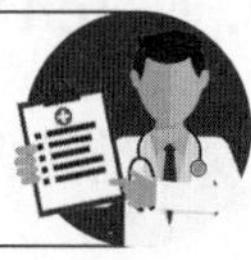

The transition to university coincides with a critical developmental period characterized by individuation and separation from family, development of new social connections, and increased autonomy and responsibility. At the same time, the brain is undergoing accelerated development

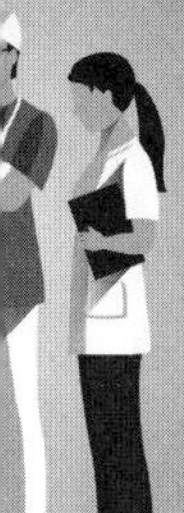

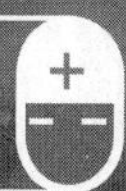

and is at heightened sensitivity to risk exposures commonly encountered by university students including psychosocial stressors, recreational drugs, alcohol binging, and sleep disruption. Moreover, most mental disorders emerge by early adulthood and are associated with a substantial delay in treatment. Untreated or inadequately treated mental illness is associated with progression to more complex disorders, school dropout, addiction, and self-harm. Taken together, the transition to university coincides with a high-risk period for maladaptive coping, onset of psychopathology, and academic failure; a corollary is that it also represents an important window of opportunity for prevention and timely intervention. Thus, universities need to take a lead role in the development of an integrated system of student mental health care.

Globally, enrolment and diversity of the university student population are increasing. A 2016 cross-national study estimated the 12-month prevalence of mental disorders in students aged 18–22 years at about one-fifth (20.3%) with anxiety being the most common, followed by mood and substance use disorders. A 2017 systematic review focusing on medical students reported a summary prevalence of 27.2% for depression or depressive symptoms and 11.1% for suicidal ideation. However, less than 20% of students screening positive or meeting diagnostic criteria for a mental disorder sought or received minimally adequate treatment.

Concurrently, universities are experiencing a substantial increase in student demand for mental health services, far in excess of enrolment increases. Focus on initiatives to raise awareness and decrease stigma may be contributing factors. Additionally, university students experience various stressors related to social relationships, loneliness, academic demands, and finances. Graduate students and those in professional schools such as medicine face additional challenges related to the intensive curriculum, heightened competition, and having to support a family while studying.

The disparity between demand and current student mental health resources has reached a tipping point. Dissatisfaction with the status quo has been expressed, highlighting inadequate student consultation in service development, inequities between programs and institutions, access barriers and gaps in services, and a need for a more complete range of responsive and evidence-informed mental health services. Community-based care is not designed to meet the needs of university students: typically a transient population who experience unique stressors during a short period of intensive study and often struggle with symptoms that fall short of inclusion criteria for specialty programs.

Several authoritative reports detailing the current state of student mental health services have made common observations: (1) academic success depends upon mental health; (2) demand for mental health services is exceeding capacity; (3) complexity of student mental health need is increasing; (4) current mental health care resources are fragmented; and (5) models of service delivery vary between institutions and none have been systematically evaluated. Notwithstanding, debate exists about the role the university should play in ensuring that accessible and effective student

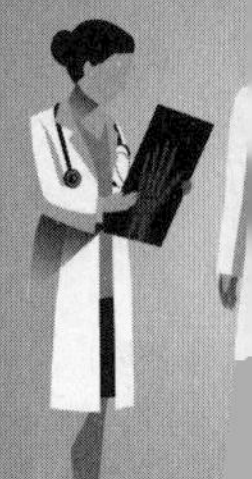

mental health services are in place to support the spectrum of mental health need.

Effective reform will probably mean reorganizing and strengthening existing services and developing new campus-based resources and facilitated pathways to community-based care. Rationalizing services along the lines of a modified stepped care approach tailored to the university environment and student population has immediate appeal. This method would reduce the risk of delay in accessing specialty treatment for the smaller but substantial number of students with emerging mental illness, while appropriately directing the larger number of help-seeking students with transient situational problems and uncomplicated symptoms to appropriate campus-based resources. Such a model could be modified to suit local environments. The success of this approach is predicated on an accessible clinical triage framework at the point of first contact staffed by experienced mental health clinicians, effectiveness of the interventions provided, and actively facilitated transitions to different levels of care when clinically indicated (i.e., stepping up or own as appropriate).

Although important roles and obligations exist that rest with multiple stakeholders and agencies, we argue that the university must take the lead in developing an integrated and coordinated system of student mental health services linked to academic supervision. The following principles should guide this development: (1) accessible, proactive, evidence-based, culturally competent, and developmentally appropriate services; (2) effective and engaging clinical triage at point of first contact; (3) facilitated transitions between campus and community-based services; (4) outcome and quality indicators embedded in routine care; (5) development of standards of care and fitness to study guidelines; and (6) integrated research to inform the development of services moving forward.

Higher educational attainment is a major social determinant of individual and societal prosperity and is predicated on mental health and wellbeing. We assert that universities have an obligation and major incentives to lead engagement with providers and commissioners to ensure that appropriate resources are in place to effectively support the sizeable number of students in need—from developing resiliency and academic support resources to crisis intervention, and timely and effective care for students with emergent mental illness.

Source: Duffy, A. et al. 2019, July 16. Mental health care for university students: A way forward? *The Lancet*.

I. Match the words with their definitions according to Passage 3.

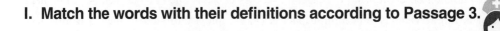

_____ 1. onset　　ⓐ a complete or wide range of related qualities, ideas, etc.

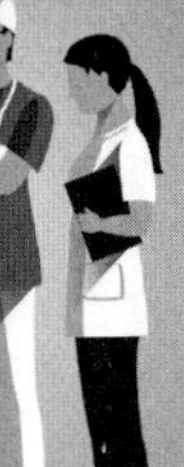

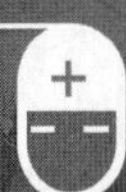

____ 2. corollary	ⓑ	to examine people in order to find out if they have a particular disease or illness
____ 3. screen	ⓒ	unfairness
____ 4. initiative	ⓓ	the beginning of sth., especially sth. unpleasant
____ 5. disparity	ⓔ	to provide people to work there
____ 6. inequity	ⓕ	a situation, an argument or a fact that is the natural and direct result of another one
____ 7. detail	ⓖ	controlling a situation by making things happen rather than waiting for things to happen and then reacting to them
____ 8. spectrum	ⓗ	a difference
____ 9. staff	ⓘ	an action taken to resolve a difficulty
____ 10. proactive	ⓙ	to give a list of facts or all the available information about sth.

II. Read Passage 3 and answer the following questions.

1. How do you understand transition to university according to the passage?

   ____

2. In what aspects are university students dissatisfied with the current status quo of mental health care?

   ____

3. What is the author's opinion on the roles of stakeholder, agency and university?

   ____

4. How do you understand the title of the passage?

   ____

5. What mental health resources should your university provide in order to keep students mentally healthy? Please give your suggestions.

   ____

III. Read the three passages comprehensively and answer the following questions.

1. What is the common theme of the three passages?

   ____

2. What is the similarity between Passage 2 and Passage 3 in terms of structure?

   ____

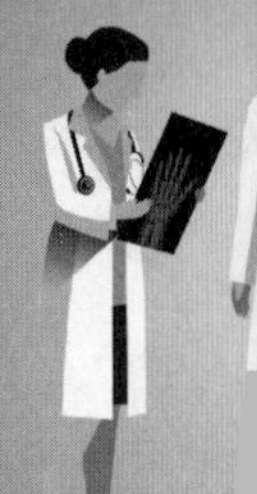

3. As a university student, how to prevent mental disorders and achieve mental health and wellbeing?

____

4. Write a short passage of about 100 words to synthesize the information of the three passages.

____

____

____

____

____

Part C Integrated Exercises

I. Read the words below, and pay attention to the pronunciation. Use the scale below (1, 2, 3) to give yourself a score for each word. Try to consult your dictionary for the words with score 1.

❶ I don't understand this word.

❷ I understand this word when I see it or hear it, but I don't know how to use it.

❸ I know this word and can use it in my own speaking and writing.

Academic words

□ address	□ adopt	□ agitated	□ artificial
□ assert	□ authoritative	□ avoid	□ burgeoning
□ champion	□ classify	□ coincide	□ commit
□ concurrently	□ conform	□ consecutive	□ corollary
□ deficit	□ deliberation	□ detail	□ determinant
□ disparity	□ elucidate	□ encounter	□ episode
□ ethnicity	□ facilitate	□ feature	□ incorporate
□ indicator	□ individuation	□ inequity	□ initiative
□ integral	□ interfere	□ minimally	□ moderate
□ notion	□ onset	□ partially	□ preamble
□ precedent	□ prevalence	□ prioritize	□ proactive
□ rationalize	□ rehabilitation	□ reiterate	□ release
□ relegate	□ resilience	□ self-efficacy	□ sensitivity

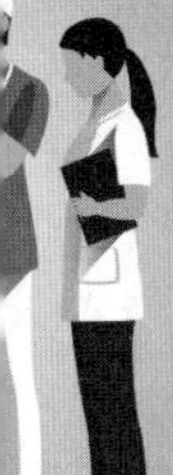

Unit 4 Mental Health

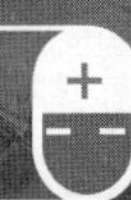

- ☐ shepherd
- ☐ spectrum
- ☐ staff
- ☐ stigma
- ☐ strengthen
- ☐ tailor
- ☐ tenet
- ☐ undergo
- ☐ vigorous
- ☐ well-being

Discipline-specific words

- ☐ behavioral
- ☐ cardiac
- ☐ cardiovascular
- ☐ chronic
- ☐ co-morbid
- ☐ cognition
- ☐ counseling
- ☐ depressive
- ☐ diabetes mellitus
- ☐ disorder
- ☐ disruption
- ☐ disturbance
- ☐ dysfunction
- ☐ hyperactivity
- ☐ incidence
- ☐ infirmity
- ☐ insomnia
- ☐ irritability
- ☐ maladaptive
- ☐ mental
- ☐ moodiness
- ☐ noncommunicable
- ☐ obstructive
- ☐ paralysis
- ☐ prognosis
- ☐ psychiatric
- ☐ psychiatrist
- ☐ psychiatry
- ☐ psychology
- ☐ psychopathology
- ☐ psychosocial
- ☐ psychotherapy
- ☐ pulmonary
- ☐ re-hospitalization
- ☐ respiratory
- ☐ screen
- ☐ self-harm
- ☐ stress
- ☐ stressor
- ☐ substance-abuse
- ☐ treatable
- ☐ withdrawal

II. Match each word in the box with the group of words that regularly occur in academic writing.

undergo	classify	reorganize	release	facilitate
encounter	adopt	avoid	commit	assert

1. ______________ one's right / sovereignty / authority
2. ______________ communication / economic growth / language learning
3. ______________ a crime / suicide / murder
4. ______________ a film / an album / an official statement
5. ______________ eye contact /conflict / confusion
6. ______________ an idea / a name / a method
7. ______________ opposition / resistance / stresses
8. ______________ the structure / the government / the company
9. ______________ data / information / documents
10. ______________ great hardship / suffering / major surgery

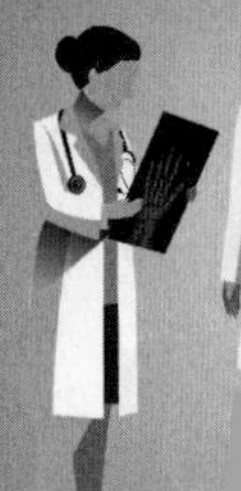

III. Study the members of the word families in the table below. Try to work out the meaning in each case according to its prefix or suffix.

The members of a word family	Chinese definitions
stress, stressful, stressor	压力、有压力的、压力源
depress, depressive, depression, depressant	
irritate, irritation, irritable, irritability	
mood, moody, moodiness	
resilience, resilient, resiliently	
rehabilitate, rehabilitation, rehabilitative	
cognition, cognitive, cognitively	
emote, emotion, emotional, emotionally	
communicate, communicable, noncommunicable	
amplify, amplifier, amplification	
incident, incidence, incidental, incidentally	
explain, explained, unexplained, explanation	
prior, prioritize, priority	
precedent, precedence, precedented	
obstruct, obstructive, obstruction	
individual, individuation, individualization, individualism	
cardiac, cardiology, cardiovascular	
maladapt, maladaptive, maladaptation	
sense, sensitize, sensitive, sensitivity	
rational, rationalize, rationality	

IV. Complete each sentence below with a word from the table above.

1. A wide range of emotionally ________ events may trigger a relapse. (stress)
2. However, elderly patients are the main group suffering seriously from ________ illnesses. (depress)
3. A lack of sleep may lead to ________ and a tendency to fly off the handle. (irritate)
4. Someone who has continuing problems after a concussion might be referred by the doctor to a ________ specialist for additional help. (rehabilitate)
5. Changes in the global climate, the environment and frequent travel to other countries led to an increase in ________ diseases. (communicate)
6. Prostate cancer has the highest ________ rate among men, and it gets a lot of attention from the media too. (incident)
7. ________ bleeding, pain and high body temperature are other possible signs. (explain)
8. Ask patients what information they would like, and ________ their information needs so that important needs can be dealt with first if time is short. (prior)
9. A thorough examination of the head and neck should be performed to look for ________, inflammation and infection. (obstruct)
10. Therapists help identify these ________ behaviors and how to counteract them. (maladapt)

V. Choose the word in each list that is not a synonym for the underlined word.

1. moderate
   A. average B. medium C. extreme D. middling
2. agitated
   A. serene B. nervous C. anxious D. upset
3. conform
   A. comply B. correspond C. accord D. deviate
4. elucidate
   A. clarify B. illuminate C. confuse D. explicate
5. vigorous
   A. powerful B. weak C. strong D. forceful
6. authoritative
   A. fabricated B. reliable C. authentic D. trustworthy
7. incorporate
   A. integrate B. contain C. encompass D. separate

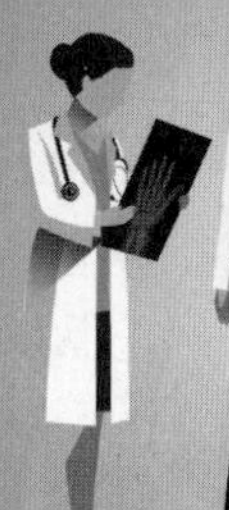

8. incentive
   A. motive B. discouragement C. stimulus D. inducement
9. stigma
   A. shame B. disgrace C. honor D. stain
10. fragmented
   A. disconnected B. integrated C. scrappy D. split

VI. Read the following expressions and sentence patterns aloud and analyze the formality of the structures used.

Target sentence patterns

1. Mental health is a state of well-being in which an individual realizes his or her own individual and collective ability as a human to think, to emote, to handle stresses, to work productively, to **interact with** each other and to **make a contribution to** his or her community.
2. The state of being mentally healthy is enviable **given** the advantages it affords.
3. **However, unfortunately**, it is a sad fact that many people around the world do not experience mental health in these ways. **Instead**, they **suffer from** different mental disorders.
4. Mental disorders are more common than cancer, diabetes, or heart disease **due to** the fact that they can affect anyone **regardless of** age, gender, social status, religion or race/ethnicity and cultural background.
5. **Put it simply**, a mental disorder **refers to** a behavioral or mental pattern that may cause suffering or a poor ability to function in life since it affects your mood, thinking and behavior.
6. Signs and symptoms of a mental disorder can vary in degree of severity, **ranging from** mild **to** moderate to severe, but mainly affect the person with it physically, socially and emotionally.
7. Socially, the person with a mental disorder may **suffer from** social withdrawal, in which they avoid or **have trouble** making or keeping friends.
8. Anxiety disorders **are characterized by** excessive worry to the point of **interfering with** the sufferer's ability to function.
9. **Despite** the fact that millions of people **are not in a position to** experience mental health, mental disorders, even the worst case, are treatable.
10. These emotional problems can even **result in** the person wanting to commit suicide or hurt others.

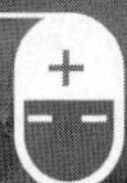

11. **According to** the WHO, mental health includes "subjective well-being, perceived self-efficacy, autonomy, competence, inter-generational dependence, and self-actualization of one's intellectual and emotional potential, among others."
12. **However**, policy continues to **lag behind** the evidence **in this regard**, as demonstrated by our global noncommunicable disease response.
13. Such a categorization would **set a precedent for** the exclusion of mental illnesses from all future WHO discussions on noncommunicable diseases.
14. We **take issue with** this viewpoint, as mental illnesses are themselves risk factors that affect the incidence and prognosis of diseases traditionally classified as "noncommunicable".
15. **In light of** this evidence, how can we possibly address the burgeoning epidemic of noncommunicable diseases without tackling co-morbid mental illnesses?
16. **As a result**, mental illnesses were featured prominently in the preambles of the Moscow Declaration, as well as in the political declaration issued by the United Nations General Assembly at the high-level meeting on noncommunicable diseases held in New York City in September 2011.
17. **To this end**, we **call on** Member States to assess and monitor co-morbid mental illnesses in primary care settings, prioritize the training of professionals in mental health care, and, critically, incorporate mental health interventions within chronic disease programs as part of a vigorous global response to noncommunicable diseases.
18. **It is not surprising** then, that in the 2008–2013 action plan for the global strategy for the prevention and control of noncommunicable diseases mental illnesses were relegated to a footnote, with the justification that they do not **share** risk factors **with** the other four types of illnesses.
19. The time has now come to **do away with** the artificial divisions between mental and physical health, as WHO's first Director-General championed so many decades ago.
20. Taken together, the transition to university **coincides with** a high-risk period for maladaptive coping, onset of psychopathology, and academic failure.
21. **Moreover**, most mental disorders emerge by early adulthood and **are associated with** a substantial delay in treatment. Untreated or inadequately treated mental illness is associated with progression to more complex disorders, school dropout, addiction, and self-harm.
22. Thus, universities need to **take a lead role in** the development of an integrated system of student mental health care.
23. Concurrently, universities are experiencing a substantial increase in student demand for mental health services, **far in excess of** enrolment increases.
24. **Notwithstanding**, debate exists about the role the university should play in ensuring that

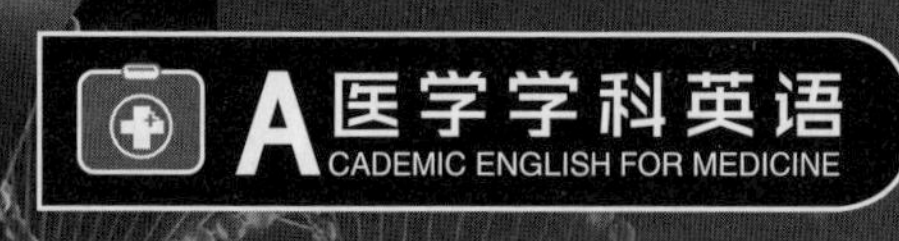

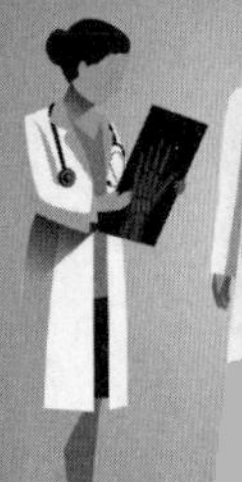

accessible and effective student mental health services **are in place to** support the spectrum of mental health need.

25. Community-based care is not designed to meet the needs of university students: typically a transient population who experience unique stressors during a short period of intensive study and often **struggle with** symptoms that **fall short of** inclusion criteria for specialty programs.

VII. For each of the sentences below, write a new sentence as similar as possible in meaning to the original one, but as formal as possible in style.

1. In short, it takes a lot of efforts for the body to break down and digest protein.

2. The characteristics of acute attacks are severe pain, swelling and erythema of the joint.

3. Smoking and drinking can badly influence your body's ability to process oxygen.

4. WHO will also be able to seek verification from States concerning reports received from sources other than the States themselves.

5. Usually we set up the infusion speed based on the age of the patient, the state of the illness, the sort of the medicine, and so on.

6. Some disagree with the idea on ethical grounds, arguing that the long-term social and emotional effects on the donor sibling are unknown.

7. For this purpose, students will write three essays about medicine.

8. As a result, treatment is often not reimbursed by insurance, for the reason that there is no "functional impairment".

9. The pressure on the hospital is much more than its capacity.

10. In spite of that, obstetric hemorrhage continues to be an important cause of maternal mortality.

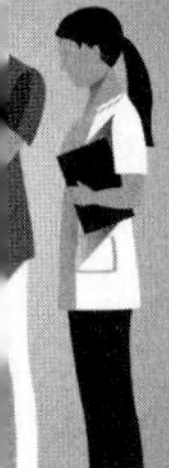

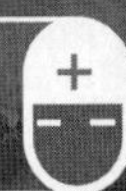

VIII. Translate the following sentences by using the following words and phrases. Make sure that your English sentences are different from the Chinese versions in terms of structures or orders, but as formal as possible. Then compare yours with your partner's according to the criteria: Whose version is more different and more formal?

1. 因为这种成分可能会与一些抗抑郁剂以及其他药物相互作用，所以请向你的医生询问后再进行添加。(interact with)

____

2. 在某些语境中，它也指代除心脏外全身任何地方的各种闭塞性血管疾病。(refer to)

____

3. 同普通的人流感一样，猪流感病情也有从轻微到严重之分。(range from… to…)

____

4. 患抑郁症的人与别人交朋友会有障碍。(have trouble making…)

____

5. 锌和铁的缺乏将导致健忘，注意力不集中，以及身体其他部分的疾病。(result in)

____

6. 鉴于本次疫情的程度以及扩展速度，加强全国各地的所有疾病控制活动至关重要。(in light of)

____

7. 维持我们体液流动的分子，其形态和多细胞生命演化的过程不谋而合。(coincide with)

____

8. 这个问题非常麻烦，因为研究证实，儿童期肥胖的孩子可能一生都要与肥胖作斗争。(struggle with)

____

9. 在反复暴发霍乱的国家应建立霍乱协调委员会。(be in place)

____

10. 研究还表明，如果你不能满足基本生活需要，就会缺乏持久的幸福。(fall short of)

____

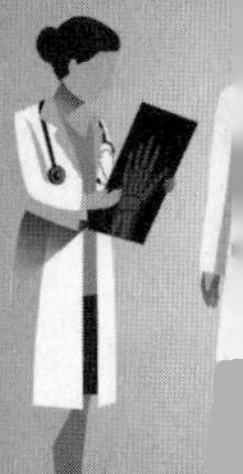

Part D | Academic Skills

Academic Listening Skill

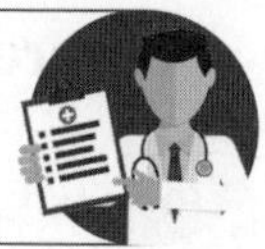

Making Predictions

Prediction is an activity listeners carry out before listening to a material. Our knowledge of the world helps us anticipate the kind of information we are likely to hear. Moreover, when we predict the topic of a talk or a conversation, all the related vocabulary stored in our brains is "activated" to help us better understand what we're listening to. If we can predict accurately what we shall hear next, our listening will be much more efficient.

While listening, it's impossible to write as fast as the lecturer speaks. If you don't have time to write down every word, you should only write down the important words in the material. Accurate predictions will help you recognize the most important words rapidly. Generally, content words are important words. They are usually nouns, verbs, adjectives, and adverbs. While these words are the most important content words, there are a few other words that are also key to understanding. These include negatives like *no, not* and *never*; demonstrative pronouns including *this, that, these* and *those*; and question words like *what, where, when, how* and *why*. Function words are not important words, which include auxiliary verbs, prepositions, articles, conjunctions, and pronouns.

Listening 1

Word bank

1. continuum	a continuous sequence in which adjacent elements are not perceptibly different from each other, but the extremes are quite distinct.
2. intervene	to come between so as to prevent or alter a result or course of events

3. upbringing	the way in which a child is cared for and taught how to behave while it is growing up
4. depression	a medical condition in which a person feels very sad and anxious and often has physical symptoms such as being unable to sleep, etc.
5. anxiety	the state of feeling nervous or worried that sth. bad is going to happen
6. contempt	the feeling that sb./sth. is without value and deserves no respect at all
7. interfere	to get involved in and try to influence a situation that does not concern you, in a way that annoys other people
8. chronic	lasting for a long time; difficult to cure or get rid of
9. disclose	to make known or public

I. Make predictions.

Before listening, think about everything you have learned and discussed about what mental health is. Write three predictions below. Compare your predictions with a partner.

1. ______________________________

2. ______________________________

3. ______________________________

II. Listen to the passage and choose the right answer to each of the questions.

❶ What does the speaker want to tell us?

Ⓐ We have mental illness or mental disorders, when we feel stressed, worried, anxious, sad, afraid or angry.

Ⓑ When left untreated, mental disorders can be chronic and long-lasting, and are associated with increased disability.

Ⓒ There are effective treatments and evidence-based interventions available, which can help individuals understand and cope with symptoms of mental illness.

Ⓓ We all have mental health which is as important as physical health. We should learn how to improve and maintain our well-being in order to live meaningful and satisfying lives.

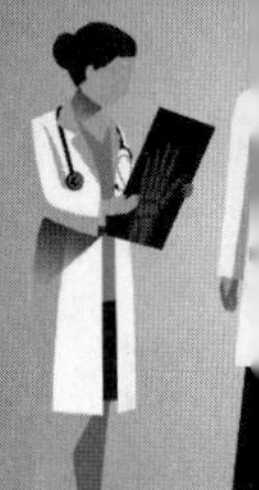

❷ **Which of the following statements is NOT correct?**

Ⓐ Mental health is as important as physical health for everyone.

Ⓑ Mental health is not restricted to mental illness or mental disorders.

Ⓒ We are on the continuum and we move up and down due to various factors such as our genetic makeup, and upbringing, our life circumstances and the stresses we are under.

Ⓓ A person is either mentally ill or mentally well.

III. Listen to the passage again and answer the following questions by filling in the blanks with the important words.

1. What is the aim of mental health interventions?

   The aim of mental health interventions is ________ the ________ so that they're able to ________ their ________ and ________.

2. What is mental health according to the World Health Organization?

   The World Health Organization describes mental health as a ________ in which every individual ________ his or her own ________ can ________ the ________, can ________, and is able to ________ his or her ________.

3. What's the meaning of being mentally healthy?

   Being mentally healthy means being ________ and able to ________, ________ in ________, being confident, feeling good about yourself, ________ and ________ your ________, ________ and ________ good ________.

4. Why do very few people with mental disorders access existing treatment services?

   This may be due to ________, such as the ________ attached to ________, the ________ of ________ of ________, ________ of how to ________ or the ________ of ________ mental health problems. Research shows that ________ remains one of the ________ from ________ for their ________ and ________ the ________ they ________.

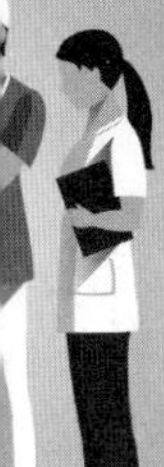

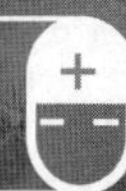

Listening 2

Word bank

1. cram	to try to learn a lot very quickly before an exam
2. cortisol	a hormone that is used in medicine to treat parts of the body that are swollen and painful
3. adrenaline	a hormone produced by the body when a person is frightened, angry, or excited, which makes the heart beat faster and prepares the body to react to danger
4. contraction	something becoming smaller or shorter
5. syndrome	used in the names of various illnesses
6. heartburn	a painful burning feeling in the lower chest caused by the stomach can not digest food correctly
7. replenish	to fill something again, or return something to its earlier condition
8. composition	the parts, substances, etc. that something is made of
9. chronic	a disease continuing for a long time
10. cytokine	a small protein produced by cells in the nervous and immune systems that affects what happens between cells
11. curb	to control or limit something that is not wanted
12. telomere	a structure at the end of a chromosome
13. chromosome	any of the rod-like structures found in all living cells, containing the chemical patterns that control what an animal or plant is like
14. irritability	the quality of becoming annoyed very easily

I. Make predictions.

Before listening, think about everything you have learned and discussed about the influences that exerts on human bodies due to stress. Write three predictions below. Compare your predictions with a partner.

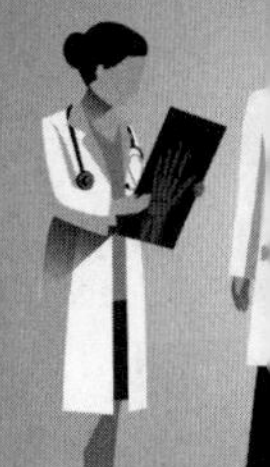

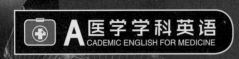

1. ______________________________
2. ______________________________
3. ______________________________

II. Listen and choose the right answer to each of the questions.

1 What does the passage mainly talk about?

A Stress is advantageous to health.
B Chronic stress is harmful to health.
C Stress exerts influences on our bodies.
D People's organs will be damaged by stress.

2 Which of the following options about chronic stress is NOT true?

A Cortisol can increase one's appetite.
B Chronic stress will immunize people against infections.
C High levels of cortisol can also cause people to put on extra calories.
D Immune system chemicals can increase people's risk of developing chronic diseases.

III. Take notes of key words while listening, and decide whether the following statements are true (T) or false (F).

1. Stress is a feeling we all experience when we are challenged or overwhelmed. ( )
2. In the short run, stress damages many of the organs and cells throughout your body. ( )
3. Chronic stress can be conductive to your health over a long period of time. ( )
4. Stress is a physical response that travels throughout your entire body. ( )
5. When your brain senses stress, it shuts down your nervous system. ( )

Academic Reading Skill

Topic Sentences

Topic sentence is a sentence that contains the main idea. On one hand, it organizes and

 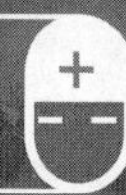

enables the development of a paragraph. On the other hand, a set of strong topic sentences will support a passage, and each topic sentence can indicate how each paragraph discusses its main idea. Unlike the topic sentence which features a "general" statement, supporting details are the "specific" statements in the rest of the paragraph. Supporting details support and develop the topic sentence, and supporting details must be relevant with the topic sentence, which will make the point convincing. Otherwise irrelevant supporting details will miss the point completely, hence a confusing passage.

Outlining is a helpful way to plan an essay or analyze it. An outline shows the point presented by the topic sentences and a list of items that support the point.

I. Look at the paragraphs below and provide an outline for them.

❶ We take the issue with this viewpoint, as mental illnesses are themselves risk factors that affect the incidence and prognosis of diseases traditionally classified as "noncommunicable". Patients with type II diabetes mellitus, for example, are twice as likely to experience depression as the general population, and those patients with diabetes who are depressed have greater difficulty with self-care. Patients suffering from mental illnesses are twice as likely to smoke cigarettes as other people, and in patients with chronic obstructive pulmonary disease, a mental illness is linked to poorer clinical outcomes. Up to 50% of cancer patients suffer from a mental illness, especially depression and anxiety, and treating symptoms of depression in cancer patients may improve survival time. Similarly, in patients who are depressed, the risk of having a heart attack is more than twice as high as in the general population; further, depression increases the risk of death in patients with cardiac disease. Moreover, treating the symptoms of depression after a heart attack has been shown to lower both mortality and re-hospitalization rates.

Topic Sentence: ______________________________

Supporting detail 1: ______________________________

Supporting detail 2: ______________________________

Supporting detail 3: ______________________________

Supporting detail 4: ______________________________

❷ The disparity between demand and current student mental health resources has reached a tipping point. Dissatisfaction with the status quo has been expressed, highlighting inadequate student consultation in service development, inequities between programs and institutions, access barriers and gaps in services, and a need for a more complete range of responsive and evidence-informed mental health services. Community-based care is not designed to meet the

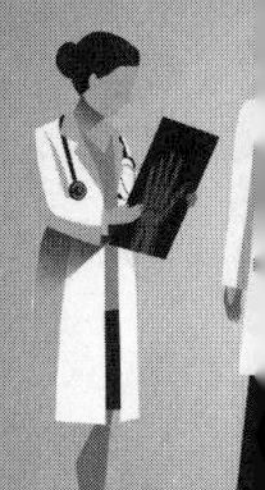

needs of university students: typically a transient population who experience unique stressors during a short period of intensive study and often struggle with symptoms that fall short of inclusion criteria for specialty programs.

Topic Sentence: ______________________

Supporting detail 1: ______________________

Supporting detail 2: ______________________

Supporting detail 3: ______________________

Supporting detail 4: ______________________

❸ As the coronavirus disease 2019 (COVID-19) pandemic progresses, a debate takes place concerning the use of masks by individuals in the community. We previously highlighted some inconsistency in WHO's initial January, 2020, guidance on this issue. Public Health England (PHE) has made a similar recommendation. By contrast, the US Centers for Disease Control and Prevention (CDC) now advises the wearing of cloth masks in public and many countries require or advise their citizens to wear masks in public places. An evidence review and analysis have supported mass masking in this pandemic. There are suggestions that WHO and PHE are revisiting the question.

Topic Sentence: ______________________

Supporting detail 1: ______________________

Supporting detail 2: ______________________

Supporting detail 3: ______________________

Supporting detail 4: ______________________

II. Only relevant supporting sentences can support the topic sentence well. Read the two topic sentences below. Then read the list of supporting sentences. Match each supporting sentence with the corresponding topic sentence by writing the number of the correct topic sentence on the line before the supporting sentence.

Topic Sentence 1: The response to SARS-CoV-2 is compromising HIV programs

Topic Sentence 2: However, social distancing is not always possible.

① ___2___ South Africa acted rapidly by imposing a lockdown, banning the sale of alcohol and taking homeless people into facilities where they could be observed and where substance-use issues among the homeless can be managed.

② ________ Many people in high HIV burden settings live in densely populated, cramped housing with limited access to sanitation.

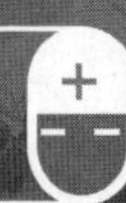

③ ________ Organizations including UNAIDS, UNICEF, and the International AIDS Society have begun to issue guidance and advice on how to deal with COVID-19 in high HIV burden settings.

④ ________ To help reduce transmission, Kenya has banned public gatherings, made the wearing of masks mandatory in public, imposed curfews, and set up isolation and quarantine centers for people who test positive for SARS-CoV-2 and their contacts, respectively.

⑤ ________ The Global Fund to Fight HIV, Tuberculosis and Malaria has also urged recipients to divert surplus funds to prepare and respond to COVID-19.

⑥ ________ As global travel and transport are disrupted; HIV drug supply chains are jeopardized.

Academic Writing Skill

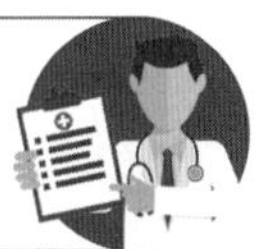

Problem and Solution

Problem-solution essays tend to be argumentative and evaluative, thus students and scholars need to convince readers that the problem is indeed a problem and the solution is reasonable. When writing a problem-solution essay, you need to explore an issue and use critical thinking to respond with solution(s).

As the following table illustrates, each component of the problem-solution structure has a specific function:

Situation	background information on a particular set of circumstances
Problem	reasons for challenging the accuracy of the figures; criticisms of or weaknesses surrounding the current situation; possible counterevidence
Solution	discussion of a way or ways to alleviate the problem
Evaluation	assessment of the merits of the proposed solution(s)

The "situation" can often be included in the introduction of an essay, and the "evaluation" may be included as part of the conclusion. Either in the introduction section or the conclusion

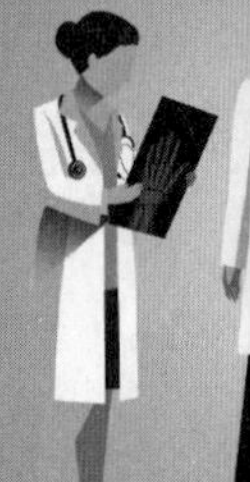

section, you can choose to state a strong thesis statement succinctly in one or two sentences as a guide map or a summary for the essay. In a long essay, you would probably have these two sections as separate paragraphs in the main part.

As the main part, the components of a problem-solution essay can be structured in two ways shown in the diagram below. For the **block structure**, all of the problems are listed first, and all of the solutions are listed afterwards. For the **chain structure**, each problem is followed immediately by the solution to that problem. Both types of structures have their merits. The former is generally clearer, especially for shorter essays, while the latter ensures that any solutions you present relate directly to the problems you have given.

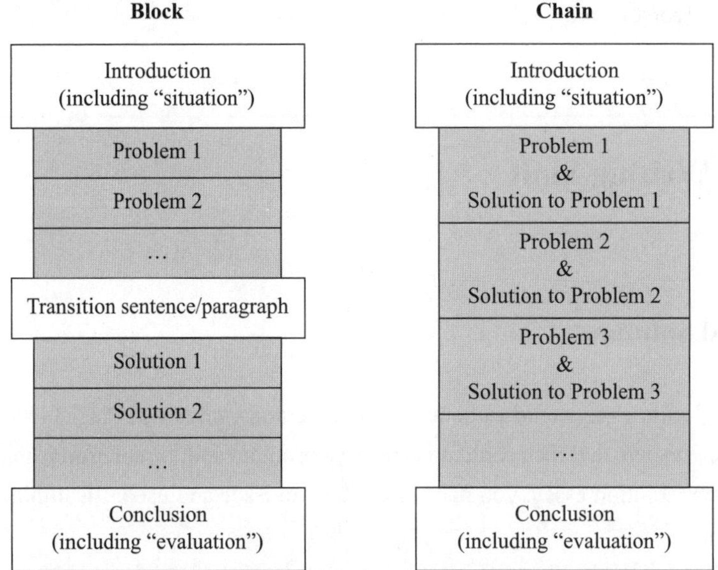

To write a convincing problem-solution essay is not an easy thing. There are several principles for you to follow in the problem and solution part.

In the problem component, you need to identify the problem and explain why there is a need to solve it. The reader's attention should be your top priority, and can be attracted by vivid description, such as staggering statistics, heartfelt personal narrative, etc.

In the solution component, when you propose a solution, you have to argue that the solution is practical, feasible, and cost-effective. Where possible, cite convincing evidence or offer specific examples for your solution(s). Organize your argument logically to make readers believe that your solution(s) will be effective.

In each problem or solution listed, you can write a **topic sentence** to state the problem or the solution in a precise manner. Moreover, you can use **signal words** to highlight the problem and solution. In the problem paragraph(s), words such as *problem/issue/challenge/difficulty/ dilemma* can be used. And in the solution paragraph(s), words and phrases like *(proposed) solution/resolve/ repair/remedy/one answer is/to solve this/to approach this/to address this* can be adopted.

I. Read Passage 3, fill in the blanks and answer the questions.

1. Introduction: Para. ________ to Para. ________

   Function: Identify the group affected by the problem and give a recommendation.

   1) To whom is the problem concerned?

   ______________________________.

   2) Why is this group of people affected?

   ______________________________.

   3) What is the author's recommendation?

   ______________________________.

2. Problem: Para. ________ to Para. ________

   Function: Analyze the core of the problem.

   1) How does the author analyze the problem?

   On one side, student ________ and ________ is on the rise worldwide; on the other side, university faces ________.

   2) What is the core of the problem?

   ______________________________.

3. Solution: Para. ________ to Para. ________

   Function: Analyze the way to solve the problem and provide guiding principles.

   1) What should be done to solve the problem effectively?

   ______________________________.

   2) What should be done urgently in order to solve the problem?

   According to the author, since ________ is the immediate appeal, the success of which is based on ________________.

   3) What is the benefit of the method mentioned above?

   ______________________________.

4. Conclusion: Para. ________ to Para. ________

   Function: Restate the solution and its content.

   1) How can university support students effectively?

   ______________________________.

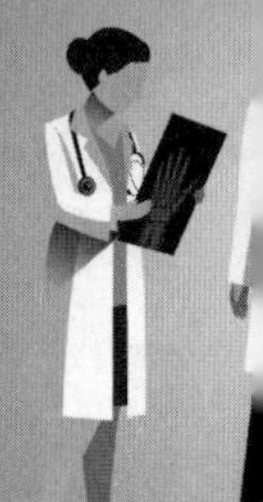

II. Below is a problem-solution essay in the block structure. Complete the essay by describing the situation, listing two other major problems, providing their corresponding solutions, and evaluating the solutions in short. The structure column and the clue sentences have been given for your reference.

Psychological Illness and Teenagers	
Introduction (including situation)	Psychological illness is very common in today's era, and especially among teenagers. Mental illnesses such as __________________ are common. More than 50% of teenagers __________________. It is a general misconception that __________________. This is not the case. Any unusual or unexpected response from an individual to very common activities is said to be "psychological illness".
Problem	Psychological illness is damaging our youth and the major reasons behind such illnesses are parental involvement, __________, and __________.
Solution 1	There are several solutions to this problem among which the following three can be very easily implemented. Firstly, parents should be better involved in the life of children. It is the utmost duty of parents to help their children rather than leaving them on their own in such a crucial situation. If a teen is in depression, the parents should bridge the communication gap, helping them release stress and face all the problems with courage.
Solution 2	Secondly, ____.
Solution 3	Thirdly, ____.
Conclusion (including evaluation)	Teenage is a very crucial phase of life and its handling is similar to that of fragile glassware. The above-stated solutions will help you in ____________________________________.

III. Now try to use the chain structure to write a problem-solution essay on the topic of mental health, and then check your writing or your peer's writing based on the following checklist.

Item	Yes or No
The essay is a problem-solution essay.	
The chain structure is used appropriately.	
The essay has a clear thesis statement.	
Each paragraph has a clear topic sentence.	
The essay has strong support (facts, reasons, examples, etc.)	
The conclusion includes a summary of the main points.	

➢ To find more information about how to write problem-solution essays, you may refer to the following sources.

1. Cynthia, C. 2018. 40 problem-solution essay topics to help you get started. Retrieved September 7, 2020, from Kibin website.
2. My Paper Writer. 2020. Problem solution essays. Retrieved September 7, 2020, from My Paper Writer website.

Unit 5

Food and Nutrient

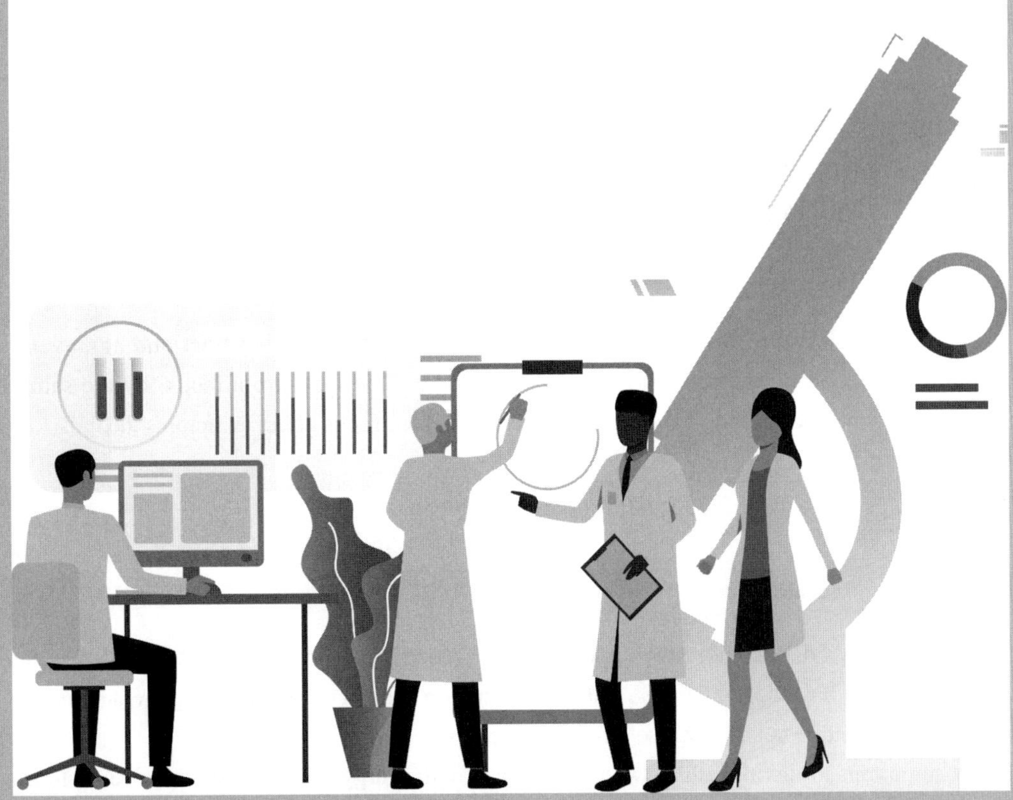

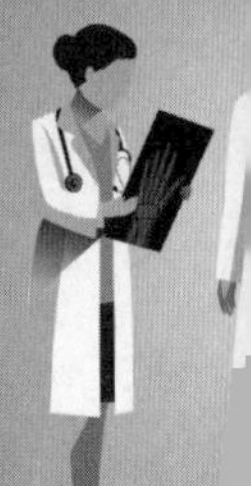

Part A | Information Searching and Delivering

I. Surf on the Internet and find information about the following topics before class.

1. food supplement
2. dietitian
3. food allergy
4. food intolerance
5. IBD

II. Make a presentation based on the information you've searched.

Part B | Text Understanding

Passage 1 Diet, Nutrition and Inflammatory Bowel Diseases (Excerpt)

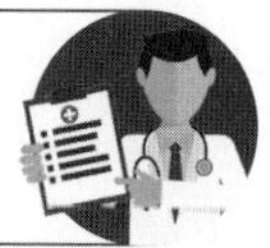

During flares, certain foods or beverages may irritate the digestive tract and aggravate symptoms. Not all people with IBD (Inflammatory Bowel Diseases) are affected by the same foods, and it may be necessary to experiment to discover which foods affect symptoms the most.

Possible trigger foods and food intolerances 

Food allergies and intolerances

Neither Crohn's disease nor ulcerative colitis is caused by a food allergy. Yet some people with IBD may also have food allergies. The most common foods causing an allergic reaction are milk, eggs, peanuts, tree nuts, wheat, soy, fish and shellfish.

It is important to distinguish between an actual food allergy and food intolerance. A food

 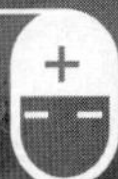

allergy is associated with an immune system response and can cause a severe and life-threatening reaction, while a food intolerance can cause GI symptoms. Many people have food intolerances—far more than have true food allergies.

Elimination diets (avoiding trigger foods) are used to determine which foods must be avoided or minimized. This involves systematically removing foods or ingredients that may be causing symptoms. It is important to do this under the supervision of your doctor and a dietitian to be sure it is done correctly without causing poor nutrition. When eliminating foods, it is important to substitute other foods, that provide the same nutrients. For example, when eliminating dairy products, be sure to obtain calcium and vitamin D from other sources.

Fiber

Dietary fiber is found in plant foods, such as fruits, vegetables, nuts and grains. It is essential for health and digestion. For many people with IBD, consuming fiber during times of disease flares or strictures can cause abdominal cramping, bloating and worsening diarrhea. But not all sources of fiber cause these problems, and some sources of fiber may help with IBD symptoms.

Soluble (ability to dissolve in water) fiber helps absorb water in the gut, slowing down the transit time of food that is stored there. It can help to reduce diarrhea by forming a gel-like consistency and delaying emptying of the intestine.

Insoluble fiber does not dissolve in water. It is more difficult to digest because it pulls water into the gut and makes food move more quickly through the gut. It is a harder and more course fiber found in the skins of foods such as apples and seeds. Consuming insoluble fiber can aggravate IBD symptoms by causing more bloating, diarrhea, gas and pain. When there is severe inflammation or narrowing, consuming insoluble fiber can lead to worsening symptoms and a blockage in the intestinal tract. Most foods contain a combination of fibers, so cooking, peeling and removing seeds are important for patients who are in a flare and need to reduce their intake of insoluble fiber.

Lactose

Lactose intolerance is a condition in which the body does not properly digest lactose, the sugar present in milk and milk products. Some people with IBD may be lactose intolerant. In addition, some people with IBD may only have problems with lactose digestion during a flare or after surgical removal of a segment of the small intestine.

Poor lactose digestion may lead to cramping, abdominal pain, gas, diarrhea and bloating. Because the symptoms of lactose intolerance may mimic those of IBD, it can be difficult to recognize lactose intolerance. Your doctor can perform a simple test called a lactose breath test to

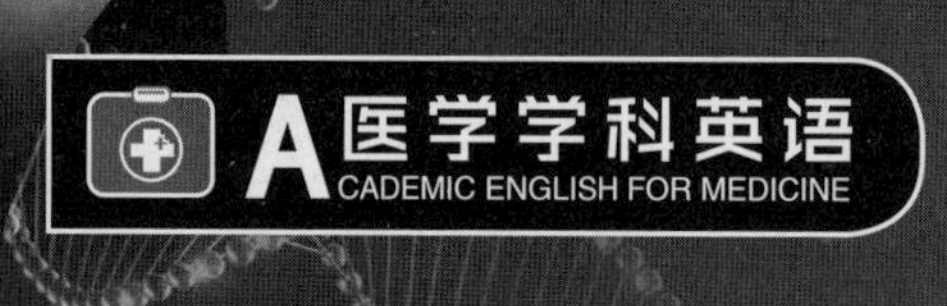

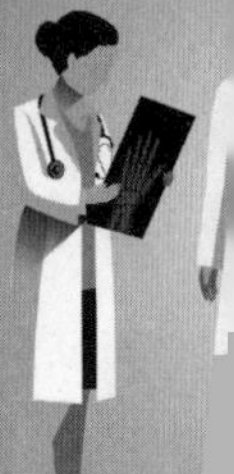

diagnose this condition. Not all people with IBD are lactose intolerant.

The severity of symptoms will depend on how much lactose an individual can tolerate. Some people may be able to consume small amounts of milk, while others may need to avoid it altogether. Lactase is the enzyme responsible for breaking down the lactose in dairy products. Lactase supplements can be taken along with milk to help digest it and specialty milk products that do not contain lactose are also available. Dairy products that contain yogurt and kefir may be more easily tolerated as well. Hard cheeses are generally well tolerated because of their minimal lactose content.

Milk and dairy products are important sources of nutrients, particularly calcium. Therefore, people who limit or eliminate milk and dairy products from their diet must be mindful about obtaining calcium from other food sources or from supplements.

High-fat foods

High-fat foods, such as butter, margarine and cream, may cause diarrhea and gas if fat absorption is incomplete. These symptoms tend to occur more in people who have inflammation in the small intestine or who have had large sections of the small intestine removed.

Gluten

Gluten is a protein found in grains including wheat, rye and barley products. Some people with IBD may be sensitive to gluten and have gluten intolerance. These people may also have symptoms of abdominal bloating and diarrhea after eating gluten-containing food, and they may benefit from avoiding foods with gluten as well. A food diary can help determine the effect of gluten-containing food on symptoms. In addition, if you suspect you have symptoms to gluten, ask your doctor for a celiac disease test. Celiac disease is an inflammatory reaction to gluten and different from gluten intolerance.

Nonabsorbable sugars (sorbitol, mannitol)

Sugar alcohols, such as sorbitol and mannitol, cause diarrhea, bloating and gas in some people. These ingredients are often found in sugarless gums and candies. Sorbitol is also found in ice cream and several types of fruits, such as apples, pears, peaches and prunes, as well as the juices of these fruits.

Source: Crohn's & Colitis Foundation of America. 2013. Diet, nutrition, and inflammatory bowel disease. Retrieved August 30, 2020, from Crohn's & Colitis Foundation of America website.

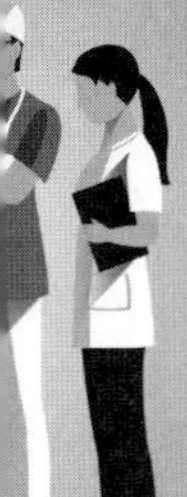

Unit 5 Food and Nutrient

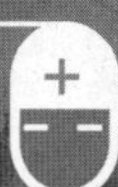

I. Match the words with their definitions according to Passage 1.

____ 1. aggravate	ⓐ a disease that causes pain and swelling in the colon, the part of the bowels
____ 2. trigger	ⓑ (of a solid) to mix with a liquid and become part of it
____ 3. dissolve	ⓒ to make an illness or a bad or unpleasant situation worse
____ 4. mindful	ⓓ a sudden, involuntary, spasmodic contraction of a muscle or group of muscles, esp. of the extremities, sometimes with severe pain
____ 5. flare	ⓔ the amount of food, drink, etc. that you take into your body
____ 6. colitis	ⓕ remembering a particular rule or fact and thinking about it when you are making decisions about what to do
____ 7. cramping	ⓖ a thick white liquid food, made by adding bacteria to milk, served cold and often flavoured with fruit
____ 8. enzyme	ⓗ an area of redness on the skin surrounding the primary site of infection or irritation
____ 9. intake	ⓘ a substance, usually produced by plants and animals, which helps a chemical change happen or happen more quickly, without being changed itself
____ 10. yogurt	ⓙ sth. that is the cause of a particular reaction or development, especially a bad one

II. Read Passage 1 and answer the following questions.

1. What's the difference between food allergy and food intolerance?

   ____

2. What are the benefits and risks of elimination diets?

   ____

3. What kind of fiber is recommended to people with IBD? And why?

   ____

4. What are the symptoms of lactose intolerance?

   ____

5. What is the function of lactase?

   ____

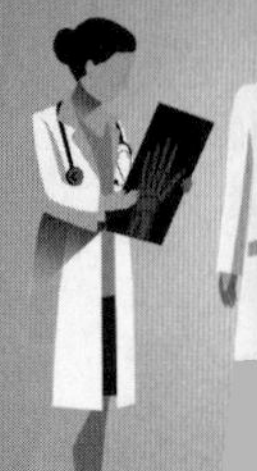

Passage 2 Fact or Fiction? Feed a Cold, Starve a Fever —The Answer Is Simmering in a Bowl of Chicken Soup

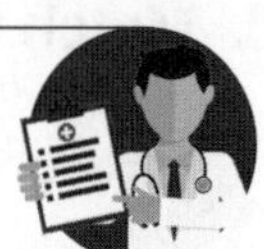

Maxims typically date back many years, but “feed a cold, starve a fever” may beat them all. This saying has been traced to a 1574 dictionary by John Withals, which noted that “fasting is a great remedy of fever.” The belief is that eating food may help the body generate warmth during a “cold” and that avoiding food may help it cool down when overheated.

But recent medical science says the old saying is wrong. It should be “feed a cold, feed a fever.”

Let’s take colds first. When your body fights an illness it needs energy, so eating healthy food is helpful. Eating can also help the body generate heat—although wearing an extra layer of clothes or slipping into bed can keep you warm, too. There’s no need to overeat, however. The body is quick to turn recently digested food into energy, and it’s also efficient at covering stored energy in fat.

The reasons to eat for fever are more interesting. Fever is part of the immune system’s attempt to beat the bugs. It raises body temperature, which increases metabolism and results in more calories burned; for each degree of temperature rise, the energy demand increases further. So taking in calories becomes important.

Even more crucial is drinking. Fever dehydrates your system, in part through increased sweating from that elevated temperature. Replacing fluids is therefore critical to helping the body battle the infection. The same is true for combating colds. “You have to make yourself drink fluids, even though all you want to do is collapse,” says William Schaffner, chair of the Department of Preventive Medicine at Vanderbilt University School of Medicine.

Dehydration also makes mucus in the nose, throat and lungs dry up, which can then clog sinuses and respiratory tubes. When mucus hardens it becomes more difficult to cough, Schaffner notes, which is our way of trying to expel mucus and the germs it contains. Staying hydrated helps keep the mucus running, which, even though it may be disgusting, is one of our natural defenses.

The challenge, of course, is that when you’re sick you may not feel much like drinking and even less like eating. Loss of appetite is common, and might be part of the body’s attempt to focus its energy on pounding the pathogens. Given the wisdom noted above, Schaffner says, don’t force yourself to eat if you don’t feel like it. “But drink,” he adds. “It’s the liquids that are important.” Avoid caffeine and alcohol. Caffeine enhances dehydration. So does alcohol, and it is also a depressant, holding us down.

What about some other common conceptions for beating colds and fevers, such as eating chicken soup? Chicken soup doesn’t possess any magic ingredients, but it has calories as well as the all-important liquids again. The warm vapor rising from the bowl can also moisten and loosen dried mucus. The same goes for vapor from hot tea, with or without lemon or honey. Taking a hot shower can soften mucus, too—and if you dare, you can get rid of it by gently blowing your nose one nostril at a time while you're in there.

Supplements are dehydrated at best. The data from studies about taking vitamin C are inconclusive, as they are for zinc. Solid studies of echinacea show no benefit. If there's any positive effect at all from any of these compounds, it is very small, Schaffner concludes.

Over-the-counter remedies may or may not help, but that's a whole another story. They can relieve symptoms but they do not kill off viruses or bacteria. Cold and fever germs usually run their course, and the immune system eventually gets the upper hand. In the meantime, drink, drink, drink. And sleep as much as you can, to give your body the rest it needs to fight the good fight.

Source: Fischetti, M. 2014, January 3. Fact or fiction?: Feed a cold, starve a fever. *Scientific American.*

I. Match the words with their definitions according to Passage 2.

____ 1. simmer	ⓐ (cause sth. to) become blocked with thick or sticky material
____ 2. maxim	ⓑ to make a person's body lose too much water
____ 3. bug	ⓒ a saying that expresses a general truth or rule of conduct
____ 4. clog	ⓓ sth. added to complete a thing, make up for a deficiency, or extend or strengthen the whole
____ 5. pound	ⓔ not certain and slightly suspicious about sth.
____ 6. dubious	ⓕ germ or infectious virus
____ 7. over-the-counter	ⓖ (of drugs and medicines) that can be obtained without a prescription
____ 8. dehydrate	ⓗ crush or beat sth. with repeated heavy strokes
____ 9. depressant	ⓘ to cook sth. by keeping it almost at boiling point
____ 10. supplement	ⓙ an agent, especially a drug, that decreases the rate of vital physiological activities

II. Read Passage 2 and answer the following questions.

1. According to the passage, what is the best way to fight cold and fever?

____

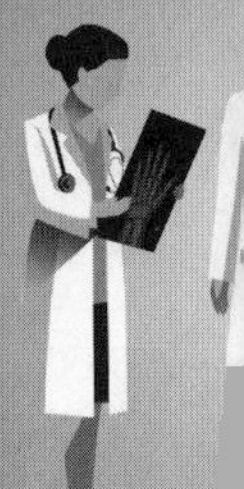

2. Why should we feed a fever rather than starve a fever?

____

3. Does chicken soup help beat colds or fevers? And why?

____

4. Are supplements like vitamin C helpful for beating colds and fevers?

____

5. Are OTC remedies helpful for beating colds and fevers?

____

Passage 3 Does Lactose Cause Bloating?

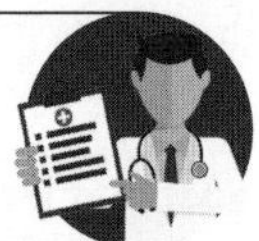

One condition that is popular among the self-diagnosis brigade is lactose intolerance. High-profile celebrities often credit their enviable figures and glowing good looks to giving up dairy (rather than airbrushing) and many of the rest of us follow suit in the hope of achieving the same results.

The trend for giving up lactose is interesting, as researchers have found that early Neolithic Europeans couldn't stomach their milk, according to the first direct examination of lactose intolerance in skeletons dating from 5840 BC to 5000 BC. Nevertheless, dairy farming persisted most probably because, unlike stream water, milk was free from parasites and safer to drink. Dairy farming became widespread and this drove the rapid evolution of lactose tolerance. This means that, today, 90% of adult Northern Europeans and some people from Africa and the Middle East possess a gene that means their bodies are able to successfully process dairy into useful nutrients.

Lactose is the main carbohydrate (known as a disaccharide) present in dairy products. During infancy, lactose accounts for most of our dietary carbohydrates. The concentration of lactose in breast milk is 7.2mg/100ml, whereas in cow's milk it is only 4.7mg/100ml.

In order to be digested and absorbed, lactose requires the presence of the enzyme lactase in the small intestine. Levels of lactase production are at a peak for around the first six months after birth, and then decline to less than 10% of that level in childhood. However, lactase activity usually persists in populations where dairy products are consumed into adulthood. These are typically white Caucasians living in Northern and Western Europe and the US.

Lactose intolerance, which can also be called lactose malabsorption or hypolactasia, is caused by low lactase activity in the gut due to a deficiency in production. Lactose intolerance occurs when the lactose cannot be digested and absorbed and then causes symptoms. Lactase deficiency has been described in three different conditions: congenital, primary late onset and secondary onset.

Congenital lactase deficiency is rare and symptoms occur shortly after birth. In the first year it is common for babies to experience partial malabsorption of lactose present in human milk or formula. This phenomenon of physiological malabsorption due to an insufficient production of the lactase enzyme may be the cause of colic. Insufficient lactase production generally only lasts for three months after birth, which coincides with the time that colicky behaviour usually subsides.

Primary late onset hypolactasia is a genetic condition that is characterized by a gradual reduction of lactase activity. Mostly, lactase deficiency manifests itself after the age of five in white populations and sometimes earlier in other racial groups. In some racial groups it does not occur before adolescence. Globally, it is the most common cause of lactose intolerance. In Europe, the frequency of primary late onset lactase deficiency varies from 2% in Scandinavia to 70% in some regions of Italy. The prevalence in the white population in the UK is at about 20%. In Asia, the incidence is close to 100%.

Secondary hypolactasia is a shortage of lactase resulting from gastrointestinal disease causing damage to the lining of the small bowel. This damage may occur as a result of various conditions such as gastroenteritis, coeliac disease or inflammatory bowel disease (Crohn's disease). Recovery of full function may take months to complete, because lactase is the last enzyme to return to normal following injury. Clinically, secondary lactase deficiency occurs after smallbowel injury, such as viral and parasitic infections. Whether it makes sense to decrease lactose intake in infants with severe gastroenteritis for a limited period of time (one to three weeks) is heavily debated, not least because breast milk, which is highly recommended for infants, contains a high amount of lactose; the general consensus is that mothers should not stop breastfeeding because of gastroenteritis. Moreover, when lactose is fermented in the colon, it results in the growth of bifidobacteria, thus stimulating a healthy gut microbiota.

The presence of undigested lactose in the colon is responsible for fluid shifts that result in watery diarrhea. Bacteria present in the colon ferment the lactose, resulting in the production of short-chain fatty acids, hydrogen, carbon dioxide and methane, which in turn cause bloating and cramps. Symptoms can increase with age, with many patients developing symptoms of lactose intolerance in adolescence and adulthood. They start shortly after consumption of milk and, although there are broad differences in response among patients, symptoms are in general related to the amount of lactose ingested. If lactose intolerance is suspected, a true diagnosis can be made using a lactose hydrogen breath test. In exceptional circumstances, this may be confirmed by a duodenal biopsy. Other measures include examination of the pH of the faeces, a blood test and/or checking for the presence of lactose in the patient's stool.

The lactose hydrogen breath test is a quick, non-invasive test that measures the content of

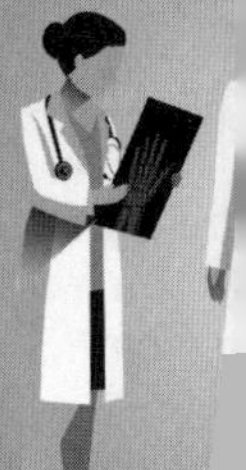

hydrogen in expired air. A high level of hydrogen is indicative of undigested lactose. The lactose tolerance blood test measures levels of glucose in the blood after a challenge with lactose. Glucose is created when lactose breaks down. For this test, several blood samples need to be taken after the intake of milk.

As for treatment, via referral, dieticians will prescribe a lactose-free or lactose-poor diet. Completely lactose-free is only needed in the rare case of infants with congenital lactase deficiency. In all the other clinical situations, some lactase activity will persist, and thus "small" amounts of lactose can be tolerated. Indeed, most people with lactose intolerance will be able to consume up to 7g of lactose (approximately 100ml of milk) without displaying symptoms. Some sufferers have even been shown to tolerate up to 500ml of milk per day. Fermented dairy products such as cheese and yogurt are in general better tolerated, as the lactose is fermented by the probiotic strains added. In many countries, lactase can be administered as an "enzymatic supplement". This exists in both powder and liquid form, and needs to be taken just before a lactose-containing meal.

Source: Westlake, H. 2019. Does lactose cause bloating?. *How It Works—Human Body Myths Busted*, 3: 23-27.

I. Match the words with their definitions according to Passage 3.

____ 1. bloating
____ 2. stomach
____ 3. concentration
____ 4. congenital
____ 5. formula
____ 6. subside
____ 7. colic
____ 8. ingest
____ 9. ferment
____ 10. diarrhea

a (of diseases, etc.) present from or before birth
b to become less violent, active, intense, etc.
c severe pain in the stomach and bowels, suffered especially by babies
d the swelling of a body or part of a body, usually because it has a lot of gas or liquid in it
e the amount of a substance in a liquid or in another substance
f an illness in which the body's solid waste is more liquid than usual and comes out of the body more often
g to be able to eat sth. without feeling ill/sick
h a type of liquid food for babies, given instead of breast milk
i to take (food, etc.) into the body, typically by swallowing
j to (cause sth. to) change chemically through the action of living substances, such as yeast or bacteria

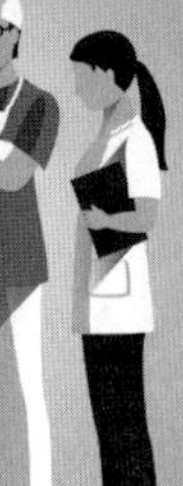

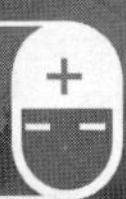

II. Read Passage 3 and answer the following questions.

1. What does the author imply by saying "rather than airbrushing" in Paragraph 1?

____

2. What is lactose intolerance?

____

3. What is the difference among congenital, primary and secondary lactose intolerance?

____

4. Why shouldn't lactose intake be reduced in infants with severe gastroenteritis?

____

5. What are the advantages of the lactose hydrogen breath test?

____

III. Read the three passages comprehensively and answer the following questions.

1. What is the common theme of the three passages?

____

2. What are the differences among the three passages in terms of topic?

____

3. In your opinion, how to avoid foods that hurt your gut?

____

4. Write a short passage of about 100 words to synthesize the information of the three passages.

____

____

____

____

____

____

____

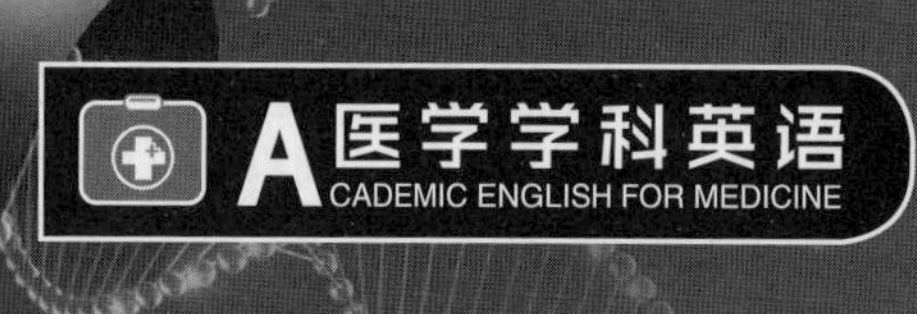

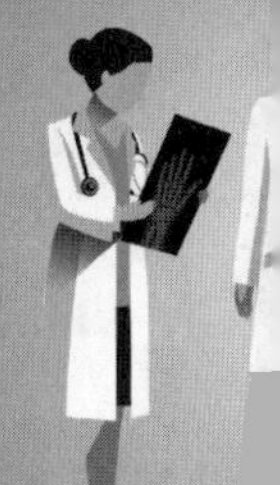

Part C | Integrated Exercises

I. Read the words below, and pay attention to the pronunciation. Use the scale below (1, 2, 3) to give yourself a score for each word. Try to consult your dictionary for the words with score 1.

❶ I don't understand this word.

❷ I understand this word when I see it or hear it, but I don't know how to use it.

❸ I know this word and can use it in my own speaking and writing.

Academic words

□ achieve	□ aggravate	□ approach	□ collapse
□ confirm	□ consensus	□ consume	□ critical
□ disgusting	□ dubious	□ eliminate	□ enhance
□ exceptional	□ generate	□ inconclusive	□ ingredient
□ insufficient	□ loosen	□ manifest	□ maxim
□ mimic	□ mindful	□ minimal	□ minimize
□ moisten	□ nonabsorbable	□ peak	□ possess
□ pound	□ relieve	□ segment	□ simmer
□ solid	□ soluble	□ specialty	□ stimulate
□ subside	□ substitute	□ supervision	□ supplement
□ systematically	□ trigger		

Discipline-specific words

□ abdominal	□ acquired	□ barley	□ bifidobacteria
□ bloating	□ blockage	□ bowel	□ bug
□ calcium	□ celiac	□ clog	□ colic
□ colitis	□ concentration	□ congenital	□ cramping
□ dehydrate	□ depressant	□ diarrhea	□ dietitian
□ digestive	□ disaccharide	□ duodenal	□ enzyme
□ faeces	□ ferment	□ fiber	□ flare
□ formula	□ gas	□ gastroenteritis	□ glucose

Unit 5 Food and Nutrient

□ gluten	□ gut	□ hypolactasia	□ inflammatory
□ ingest	□ intake	□ intestine	□ intolerance
□ irritate	□ kefir	□ lactose	□ lining
□ malabsorption	□ mannitol	□ margarine	□ methane
□ nutrient	□ parasite	□ rye	□ sorbitol
□ stomach	□ stricture	□ sugarless	□ surgical
□ tract	□ ulcerative	□ viral	

II. Match each word in the box with the group of words that regularly occur in academic writing.

achieve	replace	relieve	possess	enhance
manifest	minimize	generate	confirm	consume

1. ____________ success / balance / satisfaction
2. ____________ weakness / characteristics / symptoms
3. ____________ food / alcohol / calorie
4. ____________ death / truth / identity
5. ____________ skill / ability / productivity
6. ____________ property / wealth / talent
7. ____________ electricity / profit / heat
8. ____________ stress / strain / anxiety
9. ____________ a battery / a filter / a tube
10. ____________ cost / risk / loss

III. Study the members of the word families in the table below. Try to work out the meaning in each case according to its prefix or suffix.

The members of a word family	Chinese definitions
minimal, minimize, minimally	最小的、最小化、最低限度地
solute, soluble, insoluble	
inflame, inflammatory, inflammation	
ulcer, ulcerative, ulceration	

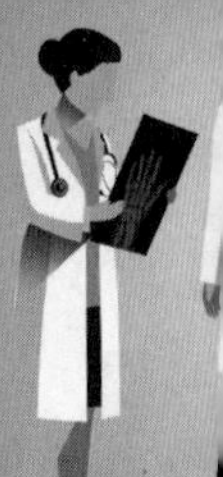

diet, dietary, dietitian	
tolerate, tolerance, intolerance	
system, systematic, systematically	
special, specialty, specialist	
nutrient, nutrition, nutritionist	
starve, starving, starvation	
elevate, elevated, elevation	
moist, moisture, moisten	
conclude, conclusive, inconclusive, conclusion	
loose, loosely, loosen	
concept, conception, conceptual	
mucus, mucous, mucoid	
gastritis, gastroenteritis, gastrointestinal	
present, presence	
absorb, absorption, malabsorption	
parasite, parasitic, parasitism	

IV. Complete each sentence below with a word from the table above.

1. ________ invasive operations are done by using small tubes, known as cannula ports, which are placed through the skin and into the abdomen. (minimal)
2. Researches showed that this kind of ventilation has many shortcomings in increasing the release of ________ factor or acute lung injury. (inflame)
3. Foot ________ and subsequent infection are a major complication of diabetes mellitus. (ulcer)
4. If you aren't sure how to create a vegetarian diet that's right for you, talk with your doctor and a registered ________. (diet)
5. Infections often lead to a life-threatening condition in which the body's immune defenses are ________ disabled. (system)
6. Death, when it eventually occurred, was probably due to a combination of dehydration,

________ and septic shock. (starve)

7. Walnut can ________ the skin, nourish the liver and kidney and strengthen the muscle and bone. (moist)
8. Researchers think daily caffeine intake can increase the risk of coronary heart disease, but the results so far have been ________. (conclude)
9. ________ hemoglobin levels thicken the blood, and the heart struggles to pump it around the body. (elevate)
10. Chronic diarrhea can be a sign of ________, which means nutrients are not being fully absorbed by the body. (absorb)

V. Choose the word in each list that is not a synonym for the underlined word.

1. <u>peak</u>
   A. summit B. bottom C. apex D. top
2. <u>blockage</u>
   A. occlusion B. obstruction C. circulation D. congestion
3. <u>mimic</u>
   A. invent B. imitate C. simulate D. ape
4. <u>solid</u>
   A. reliable B. firm C. flimsy D. sound
5. <u>ingredient</u>
   A. component B. element C. constituent D. synthesis
6. <u>segment</u>
   A. whole B. section C. part D. portion
7. <u>disgusting</u>
   A. revolting B. pleasing C. offensive D. repulsive
8. <u>stimulate</u>
   A. inspire B. provoke C. stir D. discourage
9. <u>supervision</u>
   A. monitoring B. negligence C. surveillance D. inspection
10. <u>exceptional</u>
   A. uncommon B. unconventional C. ordinary D. singular

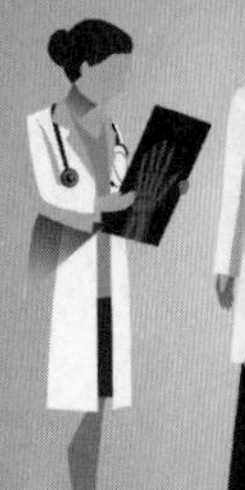

VI. Read the following expressions and sentence patterns aloud and analyze the formality of the structures used.

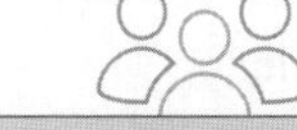

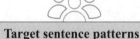

Target sentence patterns

1. It is important to **distinguish between** an actual food allergy **and** food intolerance.
2. Many people have food intolerances—**far more than** have true food allergies.
3. A food allergy **is associated with** an immune system response and can cause a severe and life-threatening reaction, **while** a food intolerance can cause GI symptoms.
4. It is important to do this **under the supervision of** your doctor and a dietitian to be sure it is done correctly without causing poor nutrition.
5. Some people with IBD may **be sensitive to** gluten and have gluten intolerance.
6. Soluble (ability to dissolve in water) fiber helps absorb water in the gut, **slowing down** the transit time of food that is stored there.
7. Most foods contain **a combination of** fibers, so cooking, peeling and removing seeds are important for patients who are in a flare and need to reduce their intake of insoluble fiber.
8. **In addition**, some people with IBD may only have problems with lactose digestion during a flare or after surgical removal of a segment of the small intestine.
9. Lactase **is** the enzyme **responsible for** breaking down the lactose in dairy products.
10. Therefore, people who limit or **eliminate** milk and dairy products **from** their diet must **be mindful about** obtaining calcium from other food sources or from supplements.
11. Maxims typically **date back** many years, but "feed a cold, starve a fever" may beat them all.
12. Replacing fluids **is** therefore **critical to** helping the body battle the infection.
13. So **taking in** calories becomes important.
14. Cold and fever germs usually run their course, and the immune system eventually **gets the upper hand.**
15. High-profile celebrities often **credit** their enviable figures and glowing good looks **to** giving up dairy (rather than airbrushing) and many of the rest of us **follow suit** in the hope of achieving the same results.
16. Nevertheless, dairy farming persisted-most probably because, unlike stream water, milk **was free from** parasites and safer to drink.
17. Dairy farming **became widespread** and this drove the rapid evolution of lactose tolerance.
18. During infancy, lactose **accounts for** most of our dietary carbohydrates.
19. Levels of lactase production **are at a peak** for around the first six months after birth, and then

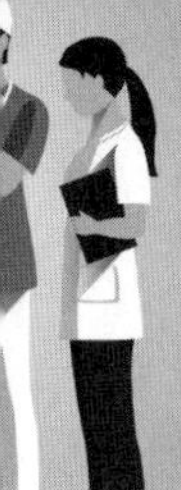

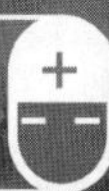

decline to less than 10% of that level in childhood.

20. Insufficient lactase production generally only lasts for three months after birth, which **coincides with** the time that colicky behaviour usually subsides.
21. Primary late onset hypolactasia is a genetic condition that **is characterized by** a gradual reduction of lactase activity.
22. Recovery of full function may take months to complete, because lactase is the **last** enzyme **to return to** normal following injury.
23. Whether it **makes sense** to decrease lactose intake in infants with severe gastroenteritis for a limited period of time (one to three weeks) is heavily debated.
24. A high level of hydrogen **is indicative of** undigested lactose.
25. Glucose is created when lactose **breaks down**.

VII. For each of the sentences below, write a new sentence as similar as possible in meaning to the original one, but as formal as possible in style.

1. Supervised by physicians, cessation rates were even better among patients who gradually reduced their dosage.

2. If you think you may be allergic to a food or drink, get rid of it from your diet.

3. He eventually died of both liver disease and a neural illness.

4. The national government will also be urged to do the same thing as other countries did with drastic measures to tackle this terrible infectious disease.

5. COVID-19 exposure notification apps become more and more popular—but will they make a difference?

6. Brittle nails indicate calcium deficiency.

7. People have been at war with germs ever since there have been people, and from time to time the germs sure take the wind.

8. Some experts owe the stress-reducing, health-related benefits of hugging to the release of oxytocin.

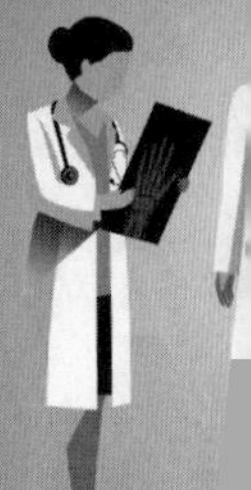

9. It was rare for any drug not to have an occasional side effect.

10. Is it reasonable to target one tumor cell chemotactic factor or its receptor when several chemotactic axes are involved in metastasis of the same cancer?

VIII. Translate the following sentences by using the following words and phrases. Make sure that your English sentences are different from the Chinese versions in terms of structures or orders, but as formal as possible. Then compare yours with your partner's according to the criteria: Whose version is more different and more formal?

1. 医生最初很难将这种传染病与流感区分开来。(distinguish between...and)

2. 女性的睡眠问题比男性严重得多，75% 的女性报告说自己有睡眠问题，而这样的男性为 25%。(far more than)

3. 我的牙齿似乎对冷和热都很敏感。(be sensitive to)

4. 这些药物是用来减缓心跳速率，其中一些甚至要终身服用。(slow down)

5. 但与此同时，治疗副作用却又可能使你难以摄取足够的热量和蛋白质。(take in)

6. 医学伦理思想的萌芽最早可追溯至公元前 15 世纪或者更早。(date back)

7. 及时的行动对维持疟疾控制进展和实现与卫生相关的发展目标将是至关重要的。(be critical to)

8. 随着年龄的增长，肌肉减少，脂肪占体重的比例增多，卡路里的消耗变缓。(account for)

9. 这项研究同时在今年的美国心脏病学院年会上公布。(coincide with)

10. 此时口腔细菌开始分解酸性物质的食物残渣。(break down)

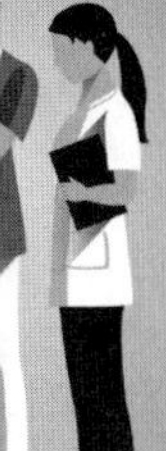

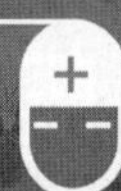

Part D Academic Skills

Academic Listening Skill

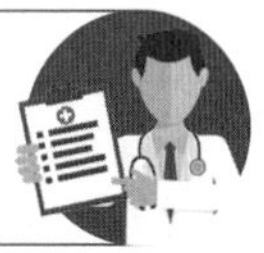

Making Inferences

In general, speakers do not always provide all the necessary information that they refer to and they only utter the most obvious pieces of information for listeners to supply as bridging assumptions. Thus, you must make inferences in order to make sense of the discourse. When you make an inference, you can use the clues given to you, along with the tone of the speaker and the knowledge that you already have to understand the speaker.

Listening 1

Word bank 

1. moderate	not very bad, small, cold, etc.
2. recruit	to form a new army, team, etc. by persuading new people to join it
3. The Mediterranean	the largest inland sea; between Europe, Africa and Asia
4. criterion (pl. criteria)	a standard or principle by which sth. is judged, or with the help of which a decision is made
5. lean	without much flesh; thin and fit
6. olive	a small green or black fruit with a strong taste, used in cooking and for its oil
7. sweeten	to make food or drinks taste sweeter by adding sugar, etc.

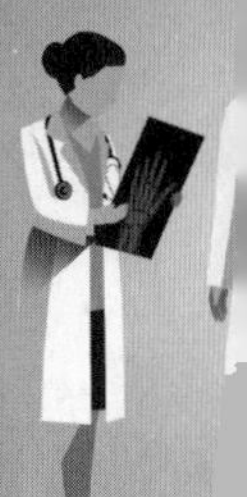

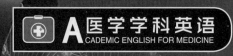

8. brutally	violently and cruelly
9. incorporate	to include sth. so that it forms a part of sth.
10. refine	to make a substance pure by taking other substances out of it
11. carbohydrate	a substance such as sugar or starch that consists of carbon, hydrogen and oxygen
12. encompass	to include a large number or range of things
13. acid	a chemical, usually a liquid, that contains hydrogen and has a pH of less than seven
14. alter	to become different; to make sb./sth. different
15. GM food	genetically modified food

I. Listen to the passage and answer the following questions.

1. Who were recruited as the subjects of the study done by researchers at Deakin University in Australia?

   The study consisted of ________ men and women with ________ to ________ ________ who had relatively ________ ________, grading each participant's ________ on a scale of ________.

2. What was the result of the experiment?

   After a 12-week study, researchers saw an average of an ________ point improvement with ________ percent ________ their mood scores so low, they no longer met the ________ for depression!

3. What on earth is a "modimed" diet?

   The "modimed" diet ________ foods such as whole grains, fruits, vegetables, low-fat ________, ________ red meat, fish, eggs and olive oil.

4. What is so special about the "modimed" diet?

   It incorporates more ________ ingredients such as olive oil and nuts while removing ________ and ________ foods such as processed meats and ________ carbohydrates. The diet is specific enough to limit sweets and processed foods while being broad enough to ________ all food groups. The incorporation of little processed oils that are high in ________ omega fatty

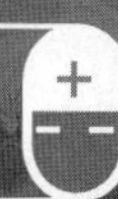

acids also aid in improving mood, especially because omega fatty acids cannot be produced by our bodies; the only source is food.

II. Listen carefully and write down "Yes" to each of the sentence which you can infer from the passage.

1. Unhealthy eating can have a negative impact on mood. ( )
2. The "modimed" diet requires people to cut down on calories. ( )
3. GM foods and refined sugars may be bad nutrition intake for the brain. ( )
4. Not all processed foods are bad for you. ( )
5. The "modimed" diet can help deal with depression ( )

Listening 2

Word bank

1. ingest	to take food or other substances into your body
2. plight	a very bad situation
3. scurvy	a disease caused by not eating foods such as fruit and vegetables that contain vitamin C
4. antidote	a substance that stops the effects of a poison
5. digest	to change food that you have just eaten into substances that your body can use
6. plasma	the yellowish liquid part of blood that contains the blood cells
7. replenish	to put new supplies into something, or to fill something again
8. pantry	a very small room in a house where food is kept
9. enzyme	a chemical substance that is produced in a plant or animal, and helps chemical changes to take place in the plant or animal
10. courier	a person or company that is paid to take packages somewhere
11. phosphorus	yellowish chemical substance that starts to burn when it is in the air, and shines in the dark

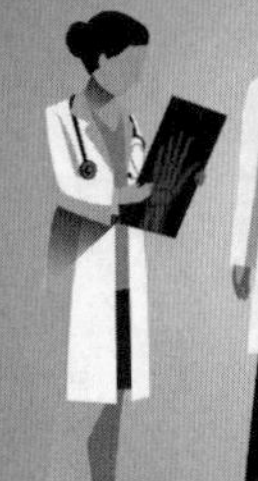

I. Listen to the passage and choose the best answer to each of the questions.

1 Which of the followings needs to be inferred?

A Vitamin C is water-soluble.

B Our bodies can't produce vitamins.

C Fat-soluble vitamins are taken up directly by the bloodstream.

D Olden-days sailors were afflicted by scurvy due to the lack of vitamin C.

2 What is the proper title for this passage?

A How Do Vitamins Work?

B How to Classify Vitamins?

C Why Are Vitamins Beneficial for Our Health?

D Why Can Vitamin A Improve People's Vision?

II. Listen to the passage and decide whether the following statements are true (T) or false (F).

1. Vitamin A helps make white blood cells and shape bones. (   )
2. Most of the water-soluble vitamins can be passed out equally easily via the kidneys. (   )
3. Vitamin C needs something that comes from proteins to act like couriers. (   )
4. If people want to improve the vision, they can resort to vitamin A. (   )
5. The more vitamin people intake, the better for their health. (   )

Academic Reading Skill

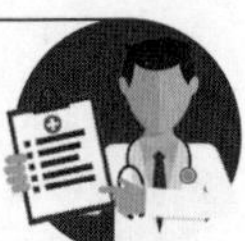

Inference Making

As an important critical thinking skill, inference making is integral to the progression in reading skills. Inference making, or reading between the lines refers to the ability to connect information across the text, bridge gaps in the information provided and draw a conclusion.

Inference making is commonly seen in daily life, from making a diagnosis from an X-ray photo to diagnosing a mechanic failure in a car. In reading, it is used to help readers understand the author's purpose, predict the causal consequence, draw a conclusion, perceive the emotion conveyed, make an evaluation, elicit main ideas and summarize the perspectives taken by the author.

One important tip to make a solid inference instead of mere guessing is attending to the evidences and hard facts mentioned in the passage. Underlying or highlighting them is a good choice. There are 4 steps you can follow to make inference. First, while reading, readers should read carefully, paying attention to the minor details and reading twice if possible. Secondly, while dealing with the inference questions, readers should understand the questions and list the applicable information you can find in the passage. Next, readers should locate the rational patterns between the details and mark the pattern and relationship between the details. Last, analyze the relations and patterns logically.

Besides, there are 5 skills readers can apply to make inferences. First, recognition of the antecedents for pronouns can help readers to connect the information consistently. Here is an example: "This involves systematically removing foods or ingredients that may be causing symptoms. It is important to do this under the supervision of your doctor and a dietitian to be sure *it* is done correctly without causing poor nutrition." If readers recognize that the italicized *it* refers to the practice of "systematically removing foods or ingredients", it will help them understand the information in a more consistent way. Secondly, as for the events and ideas presented in the passage, readers should try their best to explain them. Thirdly, it is useful to use context clues to figure out unknown words and phrases. Fourthly, readers can resort to the knowledge of the world to understand what is happening in the text. Last, offering conclusions while reading helps readers grasp the core information.

All in all, to make an inference is equally an important and useful skill, important in fostering advanced thinking skills and useful in fully understanding the passage.

I. Read the passages carefully and choose the best answer to the following questions.

1 Based on Passage 1, what consequence could it be if one gives up milk without eating supplements?

A Exerting no negative effect.
B Losing weight.
C Lacking nutrients like calcium.
D Catching some diseases.

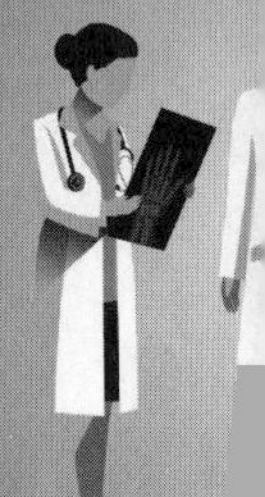

❷ According to Passage 2, what is the author's attitude towards drinking chicken soup when one catches cold?

Ⓐ Approving.

Ⓑ Disapproving.

Ⓒ Neutral.

Ⓓ Critical.

❸ According to Passage 3, which of the following statements can best support the opinion that "Colic may be caused by insufficient lactase production"?

Ⓐ Babies experience partial malabsorption of lactose.

Ⓑ Colic happens the same time when the lactase enzyme is insufficient.

Ⓒ Insufficient lactase production is common in every racial group.

Ⓓ Kids over 5 years will not suffer from lactase deficiency.

II. Read the following sentences and write down the meanings of the underlined words and phrases in Chinese.

1. Our study gives us a picture of how diet over time might be related to a person's cognitive decline, as we were able to look at flavonoid intake over many years prior to participants' dementia diagnoses.

____

2. Hepatitis A is an illness caused by the Hepatitis A virus. One way to become infected is by eating or drinking contaminated food or water. Contaminated water, shellfish, and salads are the foods most often linked to outbreaks, although other foods have also been involved.

____

3. During flares, consuming certain foods or beverages may irritate the digestive tract and aggravate symptoms and it includes consuming insoluble fiber when there is severe inflammation.

____

4. Observational studies suggest that low vitamin D concentrations might be associated with an increased risk of tuberculosis and increased mortality from the disease, but there has yet to be convincing data from a rigorous interventional trial to support vitamin D supplementation for people to prevent tuberculosis and its complications.

____

5. Babies that are born large within the normal range and people who grow tall have a lower risk of cardiovascular disease and diabetes in adulthood, but a greater risk of some cancers.

Conversely those who are born small have a greater risk of cardiovascular diseases and diabetes later in life. These effects apply not just to people who are seriously over or under-nourished, but also across the full spectrum of growth and body composition.

____

III. Read the following passage and fill in the missing sentences.

A recent study published in the journal *Depression and Anxiety* has attracted widespread media attention. Media reports said eating chocolate, in particular, dark chocolate, was linked to reduced symptoms of depression. ______________ This is because this study looked at an association between diet and depression in the general population. ______________ In other words, it was not designed to say whether eating dark chocolate caused a reduction in depressive symptoms. ______________ First, assessing chocolate intake is challenging. Then another problem is whether people report what they actually eat. Finally, the authors' results in this investigation are mathematically accurate, but misleading. This study and the media coverage that followed are perfect examples of the pitfalls of translating population-based nutrition research to public recommendations for health. ______________

A. My general advice is, if you enjoy chocolate, go for darker varieties, with fruit or nuts added, and eat it mindfully.

B. Unfortunately, we cannot use this type of evidence to promote eating chocolate as a safeguard against depression.

C. While the size of the dataset is impressive, there are major limitations to the investigation and its conclusions.

D. It did not gauge causation.

➢ To find more information about inference making, you may refer to the following sources.

1. Bailey, E. 2020. Making Inferences to improve reading comprehension. Retrieved August 26, 2020, from ThoughtCo website.
2. Roell, K. 2020. How to make an inference in 5 easy steps. Retrieved August 26, 2020, from ThoughtCo website.
3. Anne, K. 2020. Effective teaching of inference skills for reading. Retrieved August 30, 2020, from the Educational Resources Information Center website.
4. Reed, D. K. 2016. Inference making: The key to advanced reading development. Retrieved August 30, 2020, from the Iowa Reading Research Center website.

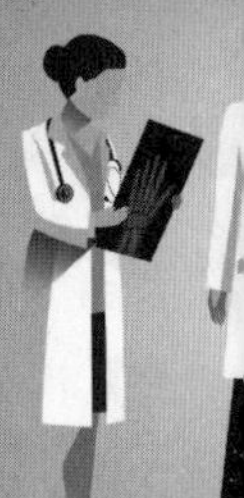

Academic Writing Skill

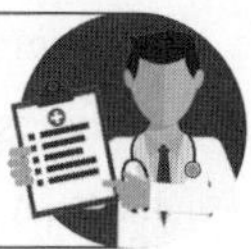

Cause and Effect

As a common type of academic writing skill, cause and effect can be used to organize a whole essay or part(s) of an essay. Cause and effect essays, sometimes referred to as reason and result essays, give reasons to the claims you make or explain why something is the case. Sometimes you can include one or more cause and effect sentences or paragraphs in your essay to support your thesis. For example, in the sentence *"High-fat foods, such as butter, margarine and cream, may cause diarrhea and gas if fat absorption is incomplete"*, the underlined part is the cause, and the double-underlined part is the effect.

As shown in the table below, there are some common signal words indicating cause and effect relationship.

Indicate cause	Indicate effect
caused by / due to as / since / because / because of owing to / be attributed to result from / as a result of / as a consequence of	cause / lead to / give rise to thus / hence / so / thereby / therefore as a result / result in / for this reason as a consequence / consequently

Correct and appropriate use of the signal words not only clarifies the relationship between cause and effect, but also puts more emphasis on one of the two sides. For example, in the following two sentences, the first sentence emphasizes the effect *(abdominal cramping, bloating and worsening diarrhea)*, while the second sentence emphasizes the cause *(it pulls water into the gut and makes food move more quickly through the gut)*.

1) For many people with IBD, consuming fiber during times of disease flares or strictures can cause abdominal cramping, bloating and worsening diarrhea.
2) Insoluble fiber is more difficult to digest because it pulls water into the gut and makes food move more quickly through the gut.

Similarly, when writing a cause and effect essay, you can adopt the block or chain structure mentioned in the writing skill of "Problem and Solution" to structure your writing.

Unit 5 Food and Nutrient

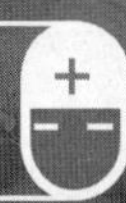

I. Read the following paragraphs to identify the cause and effect relationships, and then fill in the blanks.

1. The presence of undigested lactose in the colon is responsible for fluid shifts that result in watery diarrhea. Bacteria present in the colon ferment the lactose, resulting in the production of short-chain fatty acids, hydrogen, carbon dioxide and methane, which in turn cause bloating and cramps.

   - ______________ → ______________ → ______________
   - ______________ → ______________ → ______________

2. In some people with Crohn's disease, chronic inflammation in the intestine can cause the walls of the intestine to narrow and also form scar tissue. The scar tissue can cause narrowing of the passageway, making it difficult for digested food to pass easily through the intestine. Narrowing of the intestine is called a stricture. Dietary modifications such as a low fiber or liquid diet along with medication may be necessary if the stricture is mostly inflammatory.

   - ______________ → ______________
   - ______________ → ______________ → ______________

3. Secondary hypolactasia is a shortage of lactase resulting from gastrointestinal disease causing damage to the lining of the small bowel. This damage may occur as a result of various conditions such as gastroenteritis, coeliac disease or inflammatory bowel disease (Crohn's disease). Recovery of full function may take months to complete, because lactase is the last enzyme to return to normal following injury. Clinically, secondary lactase deficiency occurs after small-bowel injury, such as viral and parasitic infections. Whether it makes sense to decrease lactose intake in infants with severe gastroenteritis for a limited period of time (one to three weeks) is heavily debated, not least because breast milk, which is highly recommended for infants, contains a high amount of lactose; the general consensus is that mothers should not stop breastfeeding because of gastroenteritis. Moreover, when lactose is fermented in the colon, it results in the growth of bifidobacteria, thus stimulating a healthy gut microbiota.

   - ______________ → ______________ → ______________
   - ______________ → ______________
   - ______________ → ______________
   - ______________ → ______________
   - ______________ → ______________ → ______________

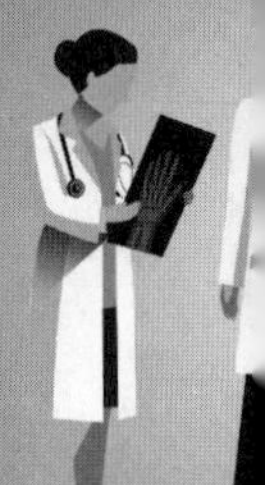

II. Write the corresponding causes or effects for the following topics.

1. Effects of eating too much junk food

____
____
____
____

2. Causes of food poisoning

____
____
____
____

3. Effects of childhood obesity

____
____
____
____

➢ To find more information about cause and effect, you may refer to the following sources.

1. Nordquist, R. 2020. Cause and effect in composition. Retrieved August 26, 2020, from ThoughtCo website.
2. White, T. 2020. Cause and effect essay outline: Types, examples and writing tips. Retrieved December 17, 2020, from Handmade Writing website.

Unit 6

Drug

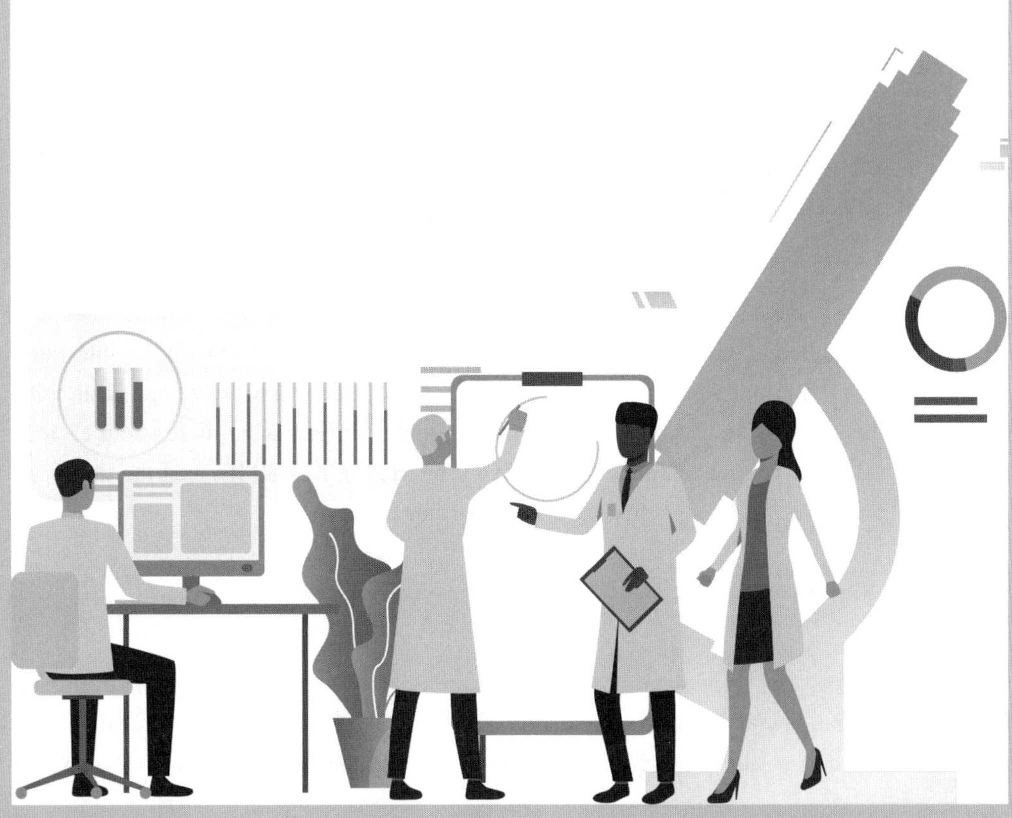

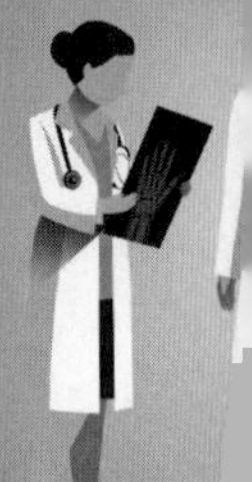

Part A | Information Searching and Delivering

I. Surf on the Internet and find information about the following topics before class.

1. traditional medicinal plants
2. chirality drug
3. route of administration
4. dosage form
5. CADD (Computer-Aided Drug Design)

II. Make a presentation based on the information you've searched.

Part B | Text Understanding

Passage 1 Medicine's Journey Through the Body

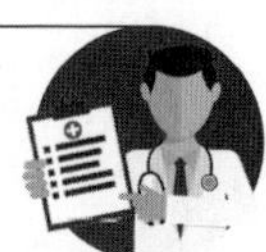

Pharmacology is the scientific field that studies how the body reacts to medicines and how medicines affect the body. Scientists funded by the National Institutes of Health are interested in many aspects of pharmacology, including one called pharmacokinetics, which deals with understanding the entire cycle of a medicine's life inside the body. Knowing more about each of the four main stages of pharmacokinetics, collectively referred to as ADME, aids the design of medicines that are more effective and that produce fewer side effects.

Absorption

The first stage of ADME is A, for absorption. Medicines are absorbed when they travel from the site of administration into the body's circulation. A few of the most common ways to administer drugs are oral (such as swallowing an aspirin tablet), intramuscular (getting a flu shot in an arm

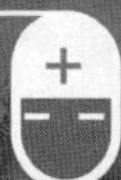

muscle), subcutaneous (injecting insulin just under the skin), intravenous (receiving chemotherapy through a vein) or transdermal (wearing a skin patch). Medicines taken by mouth are shuttled via a special blood vessel leading from the digestive tract to the liver, where a large amount of the medicine is broken down. Other routes of drug administration bypass the liver, entering the bloodstream directly or via the skin or lungs.

Distribution 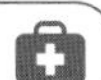

Once a drug gets absorbed, the next stage of ADME is D, for distribution. Most often, the bloodstream is the vehicle for carrying medicines throughout the body. During this step, side effects can occur when a drug has an effect at a site other than its target. For a pain reliever, the target organ might be a sore muscle in the leg; irritation of the stomach could be a side effect. Drugs destined for the central nervous system face a nearly impenetrable barricade called the blood-brain barrier that protects the brain from potentially dangerous substances such as poisons or viruses. Fortunately, pharmacologists have devised various ways to sneak some drugs past the blood-brain barrier. Other factors that can influence distribution include protein and fat molecules in the blood that can put drug molecules out of commission by latching onto them.

Metabolism 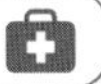

After a medicine has been distributed throughout the body and has done its job, the drug is broken down, or metabolized, the M in ADME. Everything that enters the bloodstream—whether swallowed, injected, inhaled or absorbed through the skin, is carried to the body's chemical processing plant, the liver. There, substances are chemically pummeled, twisted, cut apart, stuck together and transformed by proteins called enzymes. Many of the products of enzymatic breakdown, or metabolites, are less chemically active than the original molecule. Genetic differences can alter how certain enzymes work, also affecting their ability to metabolize drugs. Herbal products and foods, which contain many active components, can interfere with the body's ability to metabolize other drugs.

Excretion 

The now-inactive drug undergoes the final stage of its time in the body, excretion, the E in ADME. This removal happens via the urine or feces. By measuring the amounts of a drug in urine (as well as in blood), clinical pharmacologists can calculate how a person is processing a drug,

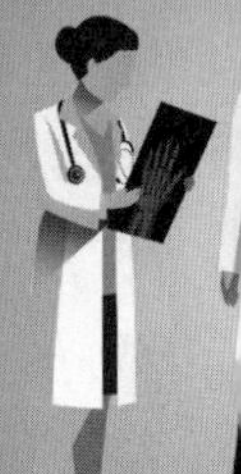

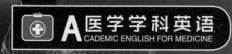

perhaps resulting in a change to the prescribed dose or even the medicine. For example, if the drug is being eliminated relatively quickly, a higher dose may be needed.

Source: Davis, A. 2014, April 30. Medicine's journey through the body: 4 stages. *Livescience*.

I. Match the words with their definitions according to Passage 1.

____ 1. shuttle	a sth. that serves as an obstacle
____ 2. route	b having no effect
____ 3. vehicle	c an established or selected course of action
____ 4. impenetrable	d to (cause sth. to) move or travel backwards and forwards, or to and fro
____ 5. barricade	e that cannot be entered, passed through or seen through
____ 6. pummel	f any of the tubes that carry blood from all parts of the body to the heart
____ 7. inactive	g a small round solid piece of medicine that you swallow
____ 8. tablet	h a medium through which sth. is transmitted, expressed, or accomplished
____ 9. vein	i to give drugs, medicine, etc. to sb.
____ 10. administer	j to strike (sb./sth.) repeatedly

II. Read Passage 1 and answer the following questions.

1. What is pharmacokinetics?

____

2. What routes can drugs be administered?

____

3. What are the factors that influence distribution according to the passage?

____

4. Why does metabolism of drugs differ among people?

____

5. Why does excretion play an important role in pharmacokinetics?

____

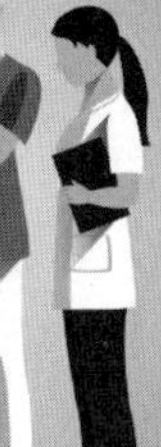

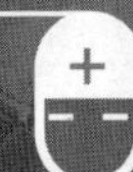

Passage 2 When Legal Drugs Harm and Illegal Drugs Help

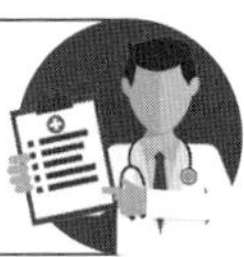

During the 1970s, the US began what has now become known as the "war on drugs", a reaction to the counterculture and drug-fueled climate of the 1960s. To the government's dismay, these policies did nothing to quell the use of illicit drugs; rather, it opened a huge market for the illegal development, distribution and importation of psychoactive and hallucinogenic substances like marijuana, cocaine, LSD and, later, ecstasy and designer drugs.

Forty years later, the US is facing a very different problem—a nation addicted to prescription drugs. And to make things a bit more complex, some of these illicit "street drugs" are now being hailed as potential breakthrough therapies for depression, post-traumatic stress disorder, and possibly even autism. With the FDA's recent decision to designate MDMA (also known as ecstasy) as a breakthrough therapy for PTSD, the increasingly blurred lines between prescription and illicit drugs in the US and their impact on health and society are becoming even more complex.

As a graduate fellow at Boston University, I helped teach an introductory course on physiological psychology. I began our section on the effects of psychoactive substances on the nervous system by revealing to my students that all bioactive substances—from caffeine to diet pills to cocaine—should be labeled as drugs, regardless of their legal status. I was met with blinking, vacant stares. Surely this perspective is not earth-shattering and most people agree that, yes, a drug is a drug no matter what label it may be attached to.

But from a sociocultural perspective, different types of drug use are associated with different, harmful stereotypes. For example, a homeless person who uses heroin is a "menace" to society but a mom recovering from back surgery who uses opioids for pain relief is just taking medicine her doctor prescribed. These problematic stereotypes have been ingrained into our culture, creating a dichotomous framework by which people understand drug use; taking (and even abusing) prescription drugs is okay because a doctor gave them to you but taking (or abusing) illicit drugs is not okay because decades ago they were placed into the illegal category.

And so herein lies our society's strange relationship to bioactive substances. Our biggest problem now lies in addressing addiction to prescription drugs, while therapeutic uses for illicit drugs are coming to light. Perhaps the greatest frustration is for those parents whose children respond only to medical cannabis to treat their epilepsy. Although there have been recent sweeping changes across the country with respect to medical cannabis regulation, and even legalized recreational use, there remains incredible confusion surrounding the legal use and transport of this semi-legalized substance.

Until there is both political and cultural alignment on how we approach the education of

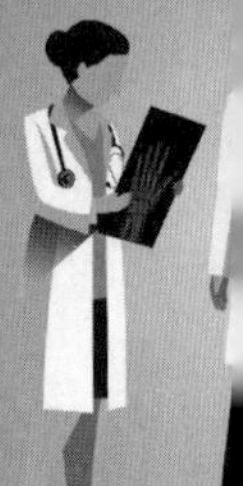

bioactive substances—what they are, what they do, and their benefits and risks—we will remain a confused and frustrated society, grasping at bits of information, or misinformation, from reliable or unreliable sources. And while many of these substances hang in the balance between legal and illegal status, we must challenge their restricted use with rigorous scientific evidence. Of course, every bioactive substance must be tested and approved by the FDA to ensure its dosing, safety and effectiveness for the intended population—but these studies require funding and support from federal resources, which they are very much lacking.

This issue can no longer be caught in a web of confusing regulations. Pioneering researchers are breaking through barriers, whether we are ready for it or not. And legislators are going to need to make decisions on these regulations sooner than they may be prepared to, starting on alignment with the FDA.

We can only hope that within the next decade the effects of the "war on drugs" will start to fade and give way to a more comprehensive and fact-based understanding of all bioactive substances. So whether you reach for the medicine bottle or the lighter, you'll understand just how each dose will affect you, the benefits and risks of consumption, and the potential for abuse—and, however you choose to use these substances, you'll have greater assistance from our health care system and a more open-minded society to support your choices.

Source: DeVito, L. 2017, December 1. When legal drugs harm and illegal drugs help. *Scientific American.*

I. Match the words with their definitions according to Passage 2.

____ 1. quell	a large and very important or significant
____ 2. illicit	b an illegal drug, taken especially by young people at parties, that gives feelings of great energy and pleasure
____ 3. ecstasy	c not allowed by law
____ 4. menace	d a synthetic drug possessing narcotic properties similar to opiates but not derived from opium
____ 5. sweeping	e to put an end to (sth.)
____ 6. vacant	f a person or thing that will probably cause serious damage, harm or danger
____ 7. alignment	g a state of agreement or cooperation among persons, groups, nations, etc., with a common cause or viewpoint
____ 8. epilepsy	h a disorder of the nervous system that causes a person to

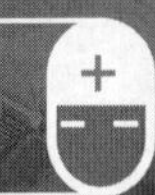

		become unconscious suddenly, often with violent movements of the body
____ 9. fade	i	to disappear gradually
____ 10. opioid	j	showing no sign of thought or intelligence; blank

II. Read Passage 2 and answer the following questions.

1. How do you understand the title?

____

2. What is the result of "war on drugs"?

____

3. Why was the author "met with blinking, vacant stares" in Paragraph 3?

____

4. What could be the future of bioactive substances in author's expectation?

____

5. What does "the medicine bottle or the lighter" imply in the last paragraph?

____

Passage 3 Dealing with Drug Pricing: Not Just One Solution

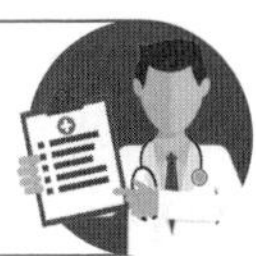

On December 11, US Food and Drug Administration Commissioner Scott Gottlieb announced a set of rules that would change the way insulin production is regulated in the US, potentially leading to increased accessibility and lower prices for the drug. Those changes will not take effect until 2020. The soaring cost and limited supply of insulin (which has been available for nearly a century) is just one example of an ongoing crisis of global drug prices, from treatments for hepatitis C that cost US $100, 000 for a single course to cancer drugs that cost $400, 000 per year per patient. According to a WHO report on global public health spending, in 2016, the world spent $7.5 trillion dollars on health, nearly 10% of the world's gross domestic product. Spending per capita on health is also highly unequal, nearly $2, 000 in high-income countries, versus only $400 and $100 in middle and low-income countries, respectively.

Drug development and dependence on curative medicine at the expense of primary care,

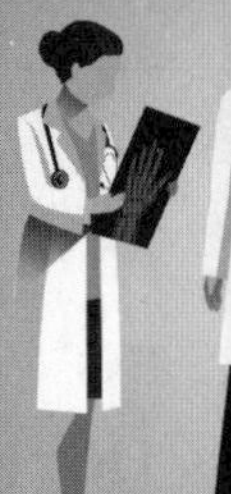

prevention, and public health in high-income countries are a huge driver of that disparity. The average annual cost of pharmaceutical spending in Organization for Economic Cooperation and Development (OECD) countries in 2016 was $573 per capita, $1, 208 in the US. An October report from University College London outlined several potential solutions. In the short term, it calls on governments to start using their powers against dysfunctional drug markets. In the US, Medicare is legally barred from negotiating drug prices with pharmaceutical companies. States can also ensure that increasing drug prices are not a one-way ratchet by using powers to legally procure generic versions of drugs, even in the face of patents, if companies refuse to drop prices to affordable levels.

Moving forward, the entire system of drug development needs to be rethought to bring the incentives in line with public health goals. Pharma companies argue that drug prices reflect the value that those drugs offer to society above alternative treatments, and that the market prices reflect an appropriate cost against the benefit that the drug provides. This argument is not entirely without merit, but ignores the fundamental fact that intellectual property rights and patent protections that allow pharma companies legal monopolies profoundly distort the market. It is impossible to say if the value of a drug's effectiveness is accurately reflected in the price, because pharma companies currently control too many of the underlying factors for the market to work. It also ignores the fact that pharma companies keep the actual costs of drug research and development closely held secrets, making quantifying the costs and benefits nearly impossible. Biosimilars have opened difficult questions of patent litigation and drugs are routinely reformulated in new, barely different guises: more than half of all drugs approved offer no additional clinically meaningful benefit.

Laws like the US Orphan Drug Act of 1983 (ODA), or programmes like Defense Advanced Research Projects Agency (DARPA), which laid the groundwork for the internet, incentivised private corporations to pursue research and development in line with stated goals, instead of just pursuit of profit. The ODA offered incentives (such as exclusivity periods and tax discounts) to companies that developed drugs for neglected diseases and proved to be an enormous success: 575 treatments for rare diseases have been approved since the law's passage, and similar legislation has been adopted in Japan and the European Union. Indeed, the ODA has become something of a victim of its own success, with pharma companies developing drugs for rare cancers under the auspices of the ODA, slicing the diseases to develop narrowly targeted treatments that are very effective for a very small number of patients, but take advantage of the benefits of the law.

The global market for pharmaceuticals is an artificially constructed one that contains innumerable barriers, restrictions, and loopholes that have developed over decades in different countries and aimed at solving different problems. Addressing drug costs will require a global effort, one that acknowledges that markets are not a panacea, and patents should not be viewed as an immutable contract. There is not a single solution to drug pricing, but any number of efforts: requiring pharma companies to offer a fair accounting of their costs, incentivising development that puts public health goals at the forefront, and ensuring that innovation is not just for innovation's or profit's sake. Some of these efforts will require serious, fundamental changes in how we approach drug development; many we could implement tomorrow, if we had the will.

Source: *The Lancet* Editorial Team. 2018. Dealing with drug pricing: Not just one solution. *The Lancet*, 392: 2665.

I. Match the words with their definitions according to Passage 3.

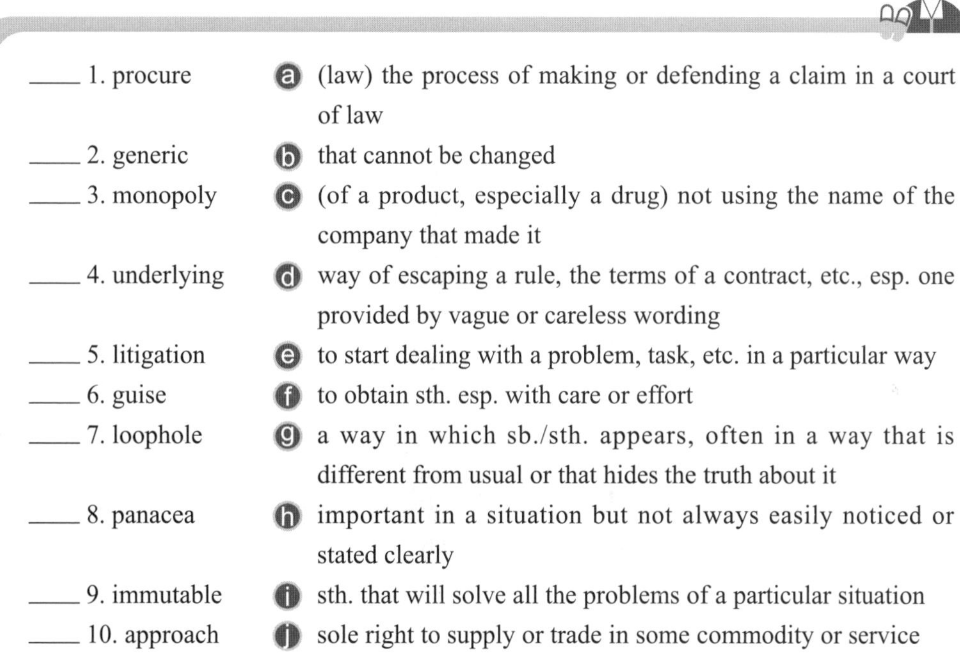

____ 1. procure	ⓐ (law) the process of making or defending a claim in a court of law
____ 2. generic	ⓑ that cannot be changed
____ 3. monopoly	ⓒ (of a product, especially a drug) not using the name of the company that made it
____ 4. underlying	ⓓ way of escaping a rule, the terms of a contract, etc., esp. one provided by vague or careless wording
____ 5. litigation	ⓔ to start dealing with a problem, task, etc. in a particular way
____ 6. guise	ⓕ to obtain sth. esp. with care or effort
____ 7. loophole	ⓖ a way in which sb./sth. appears, often in a way that is different from usual or that hides the truth about it
____ 8. panacea	ⓗ important in a situation but not always easily noticed or stated clearly
____ 9. immutable	ⓘ sth. that will solve all the problems of a particular situation
____ 10. approach	ⓙ sole right to supply or trade in some commodity or service

II. Read Passage 3 and answer the following questions.

1. How to solve the problem of drug pricing according to the passage?

   ____

2. How do pharma companies distort the market?

   ____

3. What does "a one-way ratchet" mean in Paragraph 2?

   ____

4. What could be the possible advantages of biosimilars?

   ____

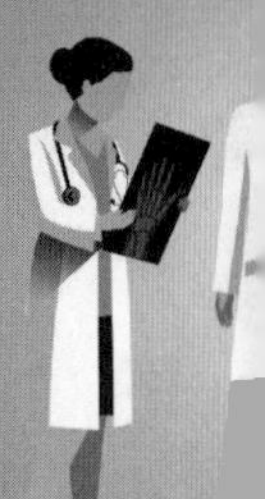

5. What are the benefits and weaknesses of ODA?

____

III. Read the three passages comprehensively and answer the following questions.

1. What is the common theme of the three passages?

____

2. What are the differences among the three passages in terms of topic?

____

3. In your opinion, how to take medications the right way?

____

4. Write a short passage of about 100 words to synthesize the information of the three passages.

____

____

____

____

____

Part C | Integrated Exercises

I. Read the words below, and pay attention to the pronunciation. Use the scale below (1, 2, 3) to give yourself a score for each word. Try to consult your dictionary for the words with score 1.

❶ I don't understand this word.
❷ I understand this word when I see it or hear it, but I don't know how to use it.
❸ I know this word and can use it in my own speaking and writing.

Academic words

□ absorption	□ accessibility	□ acknowledge	□ affordable
□ alignment	□ alternative	□ approach	□ approve
□ auspice	□ barricade	□ blurred	□ bypass

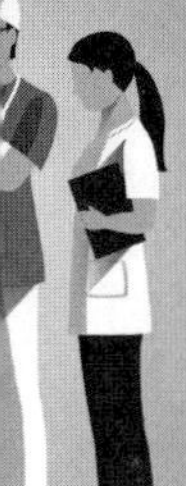

Unit 6 Drug

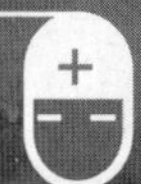

☐ collectively ☐ commissioner ☐ dichotomous ☐ distort
☐ distribution ☐ fade ☐ fuel ☐ fund
☐ fundamental ☐ generic ☐ guise ☐ illicit
☐ immutable ☐ impenetrable ☐ implement ☐ incentive
☐ ingrain ☐ innumerable ☐ legislator ☐ litigation
☐ loophole ☐ menace ☐ monopoly ☐ outline
☐ panacea ☐ potentially ☐ process ☐ procure
☐ pummel ☐ pursue ☐ quantify ☐ quell
☐ ratchet ☐ regulate ☐ reveal ☐ rigorous
☐ route ☐ routinely ☐ shuttle ☐ soaring
☐ sweeping ☐ transform ☐ underlying ☐ vacant
☐ vehicle

Discipline-specific words

☐ bioactive ☐ caffeine ☐ cannabis ☐ cocaine
☐ curative ☐ digestive ☐ dose ☐ ecstasy
☐ epilepsy ☐ excretion ☐ hallucinogenic ☐ hepatitis
☐ inactive ☐ inhale ☐ insulin ☐ irritation
☐ marijuana ☐ medicare ☐ metabolism ☐ metabolite
☐ opioid ☐ pharma ☐ pharmacologist ☐ pharmacology
☐ post-traumatic ☐ prescription ☐ psychoactive ☐ reliever
☐ tablet ☐ urine

II. Match each word in the box with the group of words that regularly occur in academic writing.

fuel	transform	regulate	pursue	acknowledge
process	implement	approve	outline	bypass

1. ______________ debate / competition / conflict
2. ______________ a difficulty / the problem / a procedure
3. ______________ an application / a budget / a loan
4. ______________ the world / the society / the environment
5. ______________ food / raw material / data
6. ______________ the business / the price / the Internet

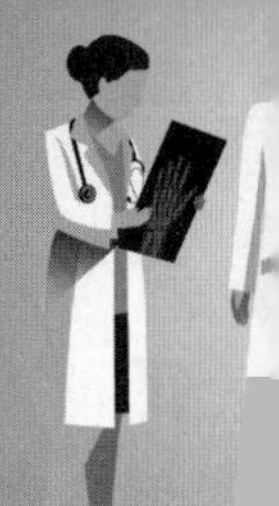

7. ______________ a goal / further study / the career
8. ______________ the framework / the structure / the background
9. ______________ reality / defeat / responsibility
10. ______________ a decision / an initiative / a scheme

III. Study the members of the word families in the table below. Try to work out the meaning in each case according to its prefix or suffix.

The members of a word family	Chinese definitions
pharmacology, pharmacological, pharmacologist	药理学、药理学的、药理学家
collect, collective, collectively	
absorb, absorbing, absorption	
relieve, relieved, reliever	
metabolic, metabolite, metabolize, metabolism	
inhale, inhaler, inhalation	
chemical, chemically, chemistry	
excrete, excretory, excretion	
potential, potentially, potentiality	
urine, urinary, urination	
irritate, irritation, irritant	
commission, commissioner, commissary	
incent, incentive, incentivize	
quantify, quantifiable, quantification	
access, accessible, accessibility	
confuse, confusion, confusing, confusingly	
legislate, legislator, legislation	
frustrate, frustrated, frustration	

distribute, distributor, distribution	
addict, addictive, addiction	

IV. Complete each sentence below with a word from the table above.

1. Vitamin D is necessary to aid the ________ of calcium from food. (absorb)
2. I think I can take most medicine except for strong pain ________. (relieve)
3. While Tamiflu is a pill that can be swallowed at home, Relenza has to be taken through an ________ and is not suitable for everyone. (inhale)
4. The medicine ________ affects your physiology. (chemical)
5. The growing tumor in the enteric cavity blocked ________ of food. (excrete)
6. Water is ideal to flush the kidneys and the ________ tract. (urine)
7. It may be that the itching is caused by contact with ________ material. (irritate)
8. It provides an easily ________ guide to all aspects of back pain and its differential diagnosis. (access)
9. Radiology was used to determine the ________ of the disease. (distribute)
10. Given the ________ power of alcohol, some women still drink heavily during pregnancy despite receiving the right advice. (addict)

V. Choose the word in each list that is not a synonym for the underlined word.

1. curative
   A. therapeutic B. baneful C. remedial D. healing
2. affordable
   A. costly B. inexpensive C. economical D. cheap
3. soaring
   A. rising B. elevated C. diminished D. ascending
4. distort
   A. falsify B. warp C. clarify D. twist
5. blurred
   A. fuzzy B. unclear C. obscure D. distinct
6. rigorous
   A. lax B. rigid C. scrupulous D. strict
7. fundamental
   A. essential B. vital C. primary D. insignificant

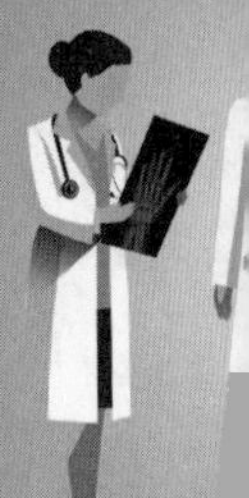

8. reveal
   A. disclose　　B. conceal　　C. uncover　　D. expose
9. innumerable
   A. infinite　　B. incalculable　　C. numberless　　D. countable
10. routinely
   A. commonly　　B. regularly　　C. rarely　　D. habitually

VI. Read the following expressions and sentence patterns aloud and analyze the formality of the structures used.

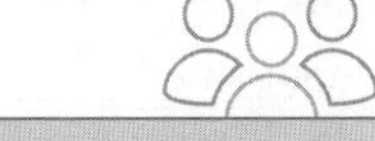

Target sentence patterns

1. Pharmacology is the scientific field that studies how the body **reacts to** medicines and how medicines affect the body.
2. Scientists funded by the National Institutes of Health **are interested in** many aspects of pharmacology, including one called pharmacokinetics, **which deals with** understanding the entire cycle of a medicine's life inside the body.
3. Medicines taken by mouth are shuttled via a special blood vessel **leading from** the digestive tract **to** the liver, **where** a large amount of the medicine is **broken down**.
4. Drugs **destined for** the central nervous system face a nearly impenetrable barricade called the blood-brain barrier that **protects** the brain **from** potentially dangerous substances such as poisons or viruses.
5. Herbal products and foods, which contain many active components, can **interfere with** the body's ability to metabolize other drugs.
6. Those changes will not **take effect** until 2020.
7. Drug development and dependence on curative medicine **at the expense of** primary care, prevention, and public health in high-income countries are a huge driver of that disparity.
8. **In the short term**, it **calls on** governments to start using their powers against dysfunctional drug markets.
9. Laws like the US Orphan Drug Act of 1983 (ODA), or programmes like Defense Advanced Research Projects Agency (DARPA), which **laid the groundwork for** the internet, incentivised private corporations to pursue research and development **in line with** stated goals, **instead of** just pursuit of profit.
10. Indeed, the ODA has become something of a victim of its own success, with pharma companies

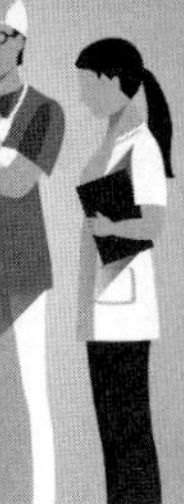

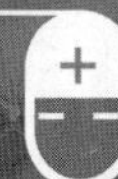

developing drugs for rare cancers **under the auspices of** the ODA, slicing the diseases to develop narrowly targeted treatments that are very effective for a very small number of patients, but **take advantage of** the benefits of the law.

11. The global market for pharmaceuticals is an artificially constructed one that contains innumerable barriers, restrictions, and loopholes that have developed over decades in different countries and **aimed at** solving different problems.
12. Addressing drug costs will require a global effort, one that acknowledges that markets are not a panacea, and patents should not **be viewed as** an immutable contract.
13. There is not a single solution to drug pricing, but any number of efforts: requiring pharma companies to offer a fair accounting of their costs, incentivising development that **puts** public health goals **at the forefront**, and ensuring that innovation is not just **for** innovation's or profit's **sake**.
14. During the 1970s, the US began **what** has now become **known as** the "war on drugs", a reaction to the counterculture and drug-fueled climate of the 1960s.
15. **To** the government's **dismay**, these policies did nothing to quell the use of illicit drugs.
16. And to make things a bit more complex, some of these illicit "street drugs" **are** now being **hailed as** potential breakthrough therapies for depression.
17. With the FDA's recent decision to **designate** MDMA (also known as ecstasy) **as** a breakthrough therapy for PTSD, the increasingly blurred lines between prescription and illicit drugs in the US and their impact on health and society are becoming even more complex.
18. I **was met with** blinking, vacant stares.
19. **Without a doubt**, male nurses receive more negative responses for doing their job than female nurses do.
20. A drug is a drug no matter what label it may **be attached to**.
21. For example, a homeless person who uses heroin is a "menace" to society but a mom **recovering from** back surgery who uses opioids for pain relief is just taking medicine her doctor prescribed.
22. These problematic stereotypes have **been ingrained into** our culture, creating a dichotomous framework by which people understand drug use.
23. Our biggest problem now **lies in** addressing addiction to prescription drugs, while therapeutic uses for illicit drugs are **coming to light**.
24. We will remain a confused and frustrated society, **grasping at** bits of information, or misinformation, from reliable or unreliable sources.
25. We can only hope that within the next decade the effects of the "war on drugs" will start to fade and **give way to** a more comprehensive and fact-based understanding of all bioactive substances.

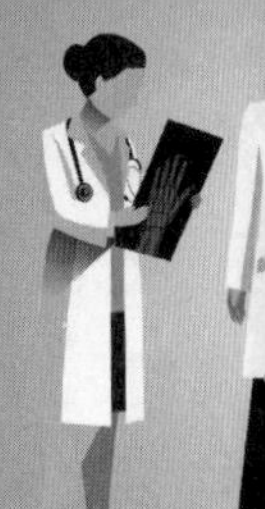

VII. For each of the sentences below, write a new sentence as similar as possible in meaning to the original one, but as formal as possible in style.

1. Putting medicines in rubbish directed toward landfill is not a good idea either.

2. Vivisection is a social evil because if it advances human knowledge, it does so at the cost of human character.

3. Starting next year, they would be banned from denying coverage to children with pre-existing conditions.

4. In addition to helping focus drug research, these findings should prepare for researchers to investigate rhinovirus evolution, diversity and drug-resistance.

5. The medical research, supported by the federal government, is being done.

6. There is no question that the human trait that sets us apart the most from the animal kingdom is our extraordinary brain.

7. In these medical attempts, we seized all of the evolving technological tools as they became available to us in our human evolution.

8. Steroid drug is honored as "major breakthrough" in COVID-19.

9. Fresh evidence has recently been known to the public that suggests this disease is transmissive.

10. Prejudice has been rooted into AIDS and changes must be made.

VIII. Translate the following sentences by using the following words and phrases. Make sure that your English sentences are different from the Chinese versions in terms of structures or orders, but as formal as possible. Then compare yours with your partner's according to the criteria: Whose version is more different and more formal?

1. 医生观察那名儿童对该药物的反应如何。(react to)

____

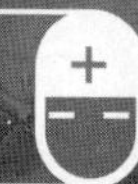

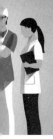

2. 药品应密封储存在阴凉、干燥处才能防潮、防高温、防火。(protect… from)

____

3. 现在处方上可以使用的大部分抗抑郁药需要数月甚至数年才能显示疗效。(take effect)

____

4. 研究表明，低碳水化合物膳食的人通常确实能在短期内降低体重。(in the short term)

____

5. 随着癌症负担的转移，一个国家的医疗水平不能再被视为控制癌症的一种障碍。(be viewed as)

____

6. 过多卡路里带来的健康风险才刚刚开始为人所知。(come to light)

____

7. 本营养添加剂能有效附着于冰鲜鱼体上，不易溶入水中造成浪费。(be attached to)

____

8. 给应急车辆让路是挽救生命的关键。(give way to)

____

9. 令他沮丧的是，尚未找到合适的移植捐献者。(to one's dismay)

____

10. 世界卫生组织会员国将 2021 年定为“国际卫生保健工作者年”。(designate… as…)

____

Part D | Academic Skills

Academic Listening Skill

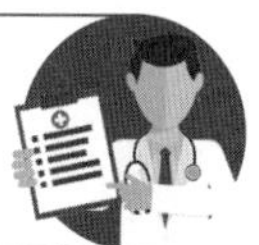

Identifying Numbers

Numbers appear very often in various listening materials. The ability of catching the exact numbers spoken in English is important. A good way is to practice the pronunciation of the numbers, particularly the difference between fifteen and fifty, etc. In addition, if a number is more than one thousand, you should mark a comma per three numbers, such as 12,000. Finally, you should note the numbers down carefully when listening.

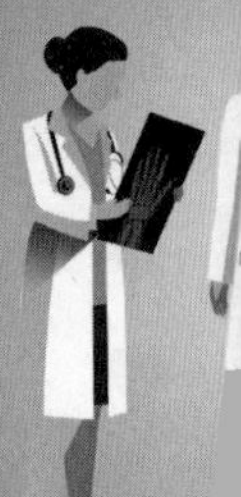

Listening 1

Word bank

1. alter	to become different
2. pharmaceutical	connected with making and selling drugs and medicines
3. FDA	Food and Drug Administration
4. preclinical	of or relating to the early phases of a disease when accurate diagnosis is not possible because symptoms of the disease have not yet appeared
5. dosage	amount of medicine to be taken at a time or over a period

I. Listen to the passage and finish the chart below.

Identify Numbers about Pharmaceutical Engineering	
Year	**Information**
From 2014 to ________	There were ________ bachelor's degrees awarded for chemical engineering.
From 2014 to ________	The bureau of labor statistics estimates the field to have a slow growth rate of ________%.
In May ________	Engineers earned a median annual salary of $ ________.

II. Listen to the passage and choose the best answer to each of the questions.

❶ **What does the passage mainly talk about?**

Ⓐ How the pharmaceutical is developed.

Ⓑ What courses a pharmaceutical engineer should attend.

Ⓒ What qualifications a pharmaceutical engineer should have.

Ⓓ How to be a pharmaceutical engineer and what jobs he/she would accomplish.

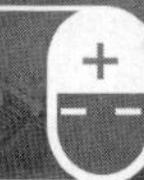

❷ **Which of the following options is NOT correct?**

Ⓐ Preclinical studies must be performed before a drug is marketed.

Ⓑ From 2014 to 2020, the number of pharmaceutical engineers is on the decline.

Ⓒ If one person aspires to be a pharmaceutical engineer, he/she needs to hold a master's degree.

Ⓓ Top undergraduate schools for chemical engineering include MIT, UC Berkeley, Georgia Institute of Technology and Stanford.

Listening 2

Word bank

1. ibuprofen	a drug used to reduce pain and inflammation
2. sprain	to injure a joint in your body, especially your wrist or ankle, by suddenly twisting it
3. hitch	to get a free ride in a person's car
4. snare	to catch sth.
5. neutralize	to counteract the activity or effect of make ineffective
6. disintegrate	to break into small parts or pieces and be destroyed
7. enzyme	a substance, produced by all living things, which helps a chemical change happen or happen more quickly, without being changed itself
8. metabolite	any substance involved in metabolism (either as a product of metabolism or as necessary for metabolism)
9. unscathed	not hurt
10. bind	to tie sb./sth. with rope, string, etc.
11. loop	a shape like a curve or circle made by a line curving right round and crossing itself
12. fraction	a small part or amount of sth.
13. fluctuate	to change frequently in size, amount, quality, etc., especially from one extreme to another

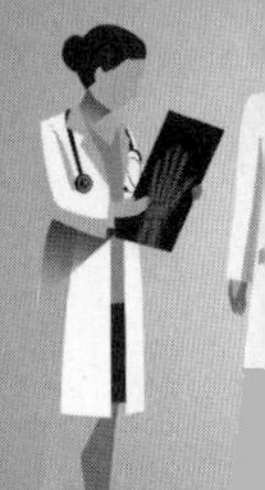

14. bet	the thing or course of action that they should choose
15. pharmacist	a person whose job is to prepare medicines and sell or give them to the public in a shop/store or in a hospital

I. Listen to the passage and choose the best answer to each of the questions.

1 How does a painkiller get where it needs to go?

A Through the liver.
B Through the circulatory bloodstream.
C Through the kidney.
D Through the small intestine.

2 Why is it so hard to get the right dosage?

A Because some patients don't listen to their doctors or pharmacists.
B Because some patients don't read the label.
C Because a lot of factors will influence the body's efficiency of processing medicine.
D Because the level of liver enzymes that neutralize medication highly fluctuates.

II. Listen carefully and then write down the route of ibuprofen in our body.

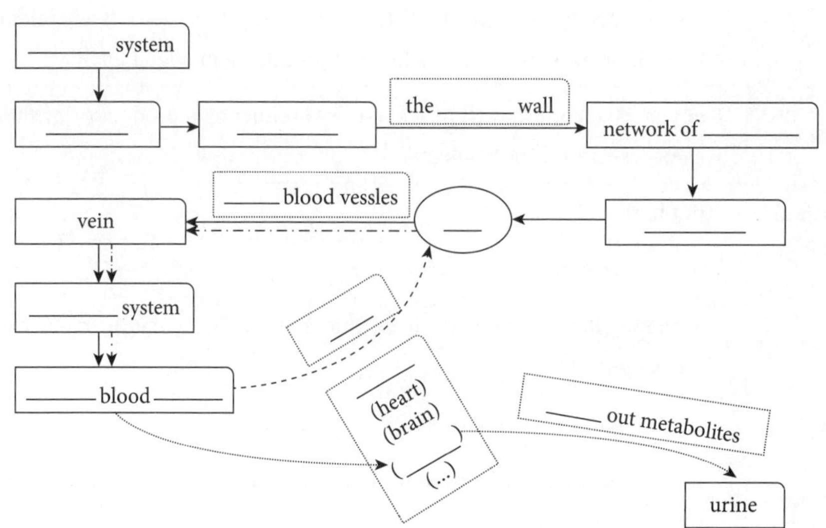

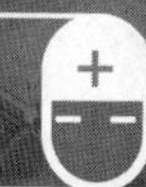

Unit 6 Drug

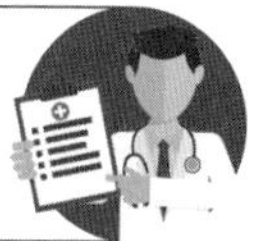

Academic Reading Skill

Facts and Opinions

Fact and opinion are commonly seen in academic paper, and they are mostly interwoven in the passage to serve the purposes of writing: to explore ideas, to persuade, to explain, to solve problems, to argue or to inform. To train our critical and analytical skills and heighten our research skills, it is important to tell fact from opinion in any passage where fact and opinion are mixed together.

To tell them apart, we should know what fact and opinion respectively refer to and their differences. Fact is often defined as something true or verified, often backed with evidences, while opinion is something people believe or think about, like personal belief. They are different in several aspects. (1) Fact is based on observation or research while opinion is based on assumption or personal view. (2) Fact is objective while opinion is subjective. (3) Fact is not debatable while opinion can be argued and debated.

Besides, knowing signal words and phrases turns out to be a good way for us to distinguish fact from opinion. Words and phrases like *demonstrate, confirm, discover, according to* are often in conjunction with fact, while words reflecting one's judgment and opinion, some modal words and phrases, such as *claim, view, argue, suspect, agree,* are used to introduce opinion.

In a nutshell, while reading, we can take advantage of the signal words, and phrases to distinguish fact from opinion, so as to unravel the thread of what is true from what is belief.

I. Read the statements below and mark with F (fact) or O (opinion) on the line before each statement.

1. ________ Other routes of drug administration bypass the liver, entering the bloodstream directly or via the skin or lungs.
2. ________ Other factors that can influence distribution include protein and fat molecules in the blood that can put drug molecules out of commission by latching onto them.
3. ________ According to a WHO report on global public health spending, in 2016, the world spent \$7.5 trillion dollars on health, nearly 10% of the world's gross domestic product.
4. ________ Moving forward, the entire system of drug development needs to be rethought to bring the incentives in line with public health goals.

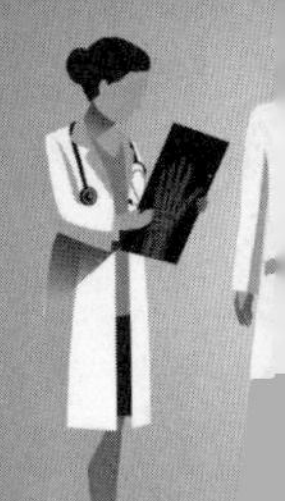

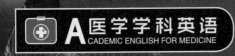

5. ________ This argument is not entirely without merit, but ignores the fundamental fact that intellectual property rights and patent protections that allow pharma companies legal monopolies profoundly distort the market.
6. ________ The ODA offered incentives to companies that developed drugs for neglected diseases.
7. ________ Addressing drug costs will require a global effort, one that acknowledges that markets are not a panacea, and patents should not be viewed as an immutable contract.
8. ________ But from a sociocultural perspective, different types of drug use are associated with different, harmful stereotypes.
9. ________ Perhaps the greatest frustration is for those parents whose children respond only to medical cannabis to treat their epilepsy.
10. ________ Until there is both political and cultural alignment on how we approach the education of bioactive substances, we will remain a confused and frustrated society, grasping at bits of information, or misinformation, from reliable or unreliable sources.

II. Read the passage below and complete the following tasks.

We're now working on 3D simulations of the heart to explore drug cardiac safety and efficacy on a larger scale. It includes an exploration of diseased conditions, such as acute ischemia—where the blood flow in one of the arteries around the heart is obstructed. This research is also part of the European CompBioMed project to build computer models for the whole human body: a virtual human. By bringing together academia, the pharmaceutical industry and regulatory agencies, we hope to accelerate the uptake of human-based in silico methodologies for the evaluation of cardiac drug safety and efficacy. Computer simulations are a faster, cheaper and effective alternative to animal experiments and they will soon play an important role in the early stages of drug development.

❶ Has 3D simulation been studied to explore drug heart safety and efficacy on a larger scale?

Ⓐ Yes. Ⓑ No. Ⓒ Not mentioned.

❷ Has the uptake of human-based in silico methodologies been accelerated?

Ⓐ Yes. Ⓑ No. Ⓒ Not mentioned.

❸ Will computer simulation play an important role in the early stages of drug development?

Ⓐ Yes. Ⓑ No. Ⓒ Not mentioned.

❹ List out the signal words that introduce opinions.

____

➢ To find more information about how to distinguish between fact and opinion, you may refer to the following sources.

1. ICOSA Project, Language Centre, HKBU. 2013. Reading skills 2— differentiating fact from opinion. Retrieved August 30, 2020, from ICOSA Project, Language Centre, HKBU website.
2. Surbhi, S. 2017. Difference between fact and opinion. Retrieved August 30, 2020, from keydifferences website.

Academic Writing Skill

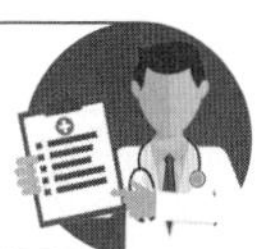

Examples and Statistics

When writing an essay, examples and statistics can be persuasive and powerful components to support what you're trying to prove in the paragraphs. Hence, the ability to provide examples and statistics appropriately and effectively is essential to successful writing.

Appropriate and effective examples must be well-chosen to add more information to explain, persuade, define, or illustrate a general idea. Not only do they provide solid support and strong evidence, but the vivid description they often include helps to capture and retain the reader's attention. You'd better ask yourself two questions before using the examples: Do these examples support my thesis? Are they relevant, adequate, and convincing enough?

An example can be organized in your writing as a case *(e.g. This has been seen **in the case of**...)*; as the main information in a sentence *(e.g. **For example**, the word "doctor" used to mean a "learned man".)*; or as additional information in a sentence *(e.g. Many diseases can result at least in part from stress, **including**: arthritis, asthma, and migraine.)*. The common signal words for exemplifying are *for example, for instance, to illustrate, to give an example, take...for example, such as, namely, including...*

Statistics convey information in numerical form (often referred to as data), such as percentages, averages, ranges, proportions, trends, and so forth. Be sure that your statistics come from authoritative and factual sources.

Include the same-topic-statistics in the same paragraph or section, and present your statistics in a clear and straightforward way instead of an ambiguous manner when you write with statistics. The following sentence patterns are often employed to present statistics:

Used to describe percentages	More than half/50% of… that…
	Of the… nearly one-third… that…
Used to describe averages	The average of… is…
	The mean score for the… was…
Used to describe ranges	… lies in the range of…
	… range from… to…
Used to describe proportions	… has the highest/lowest proportion of…
	The proportion of… reached…
Used to describe trends	The number of… has increased/decreased…
	The numbers show a steady increase/decrease from… to…
Used to compare	This finding is consistent with… that…
	Compared with…
Used to infer a broader sense	The statistics show/demonstrate/suggest that…
	Taking into account the statistical data, we can infer that…

After you introduce statistics into your writing, in order to support the argument effectively, you must connect the statistics with your argument (supporting or opposing) through explanation, organization, transition, etc.

I. Writing an essay titled "Physical Activity and Cancer" by taking the following steps:

a) Select available statistics and examples from the pictures below.
b) Build your argument.
c) Present the statistics and examples in complete sentences.
(E.g. Many studies have found that there is a strong link between being physically active and a decreased risk of colon cancer. According to JAMA Internal Medicine, physically active individuals have a 16% lower risk of colon cancer than the inactive ones.)
d) Incorporate them into the writing to support your argument.
e) End your writing with a strong conclusion to restate your position.

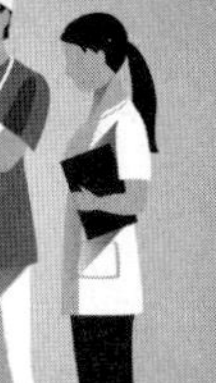

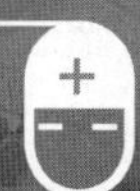

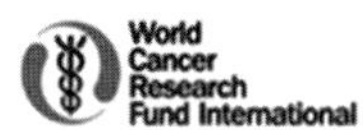

World Cancer Research Fund International

Obesity, physical activity and cancer

There is a strong link between being overweight or obese & an **increased risk** of 10 cancers:

- Liver
- Advanced prostate
- Ovarian
- Gallbladder
- Kidney
- Colorectal (bowel)
- Oesophageal*
- Postmenopausal breast
- Pancreatic
- Endometrial (womb)

1.9 billion adults worldwide are overweight or obese. This exceeds the population of China

Physical inactivity is the 4th leading cause of death worldwide

There is a strong link between being physically active & a **decreased risk** of 3 cancers:

- Postmenopausal breast
- Colorectal (bowel)
- Endometrial (womb)

Top 10 countries* with the highest % of overweight or obese adults

- Mexico 71.3%
- United States 68.6%
- Chile 64.5%
- New Zealand 63.8%
- Australia 63.4%
- Israel 62.2%
- United Kingdom 61.9%
- Hungary 61.6%
- Ireland 61%
- Finland 59.2%
- Luxembourg 59.2%

www.wcrf.org

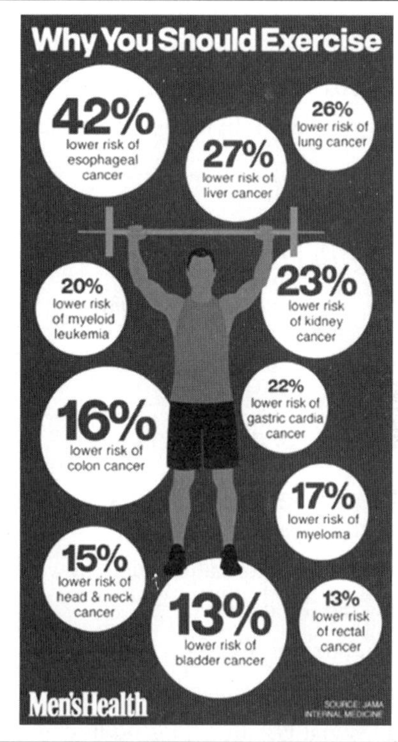

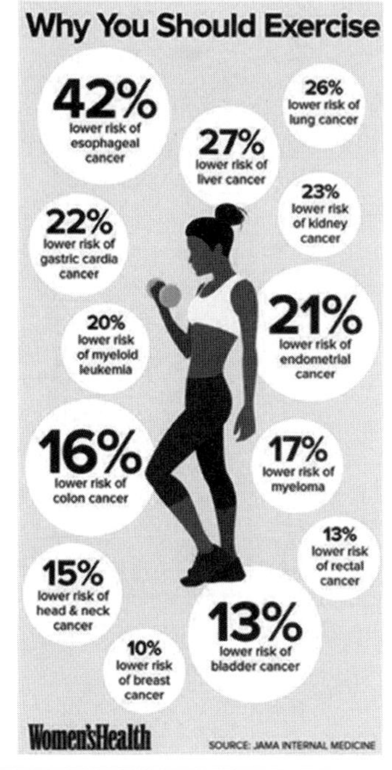

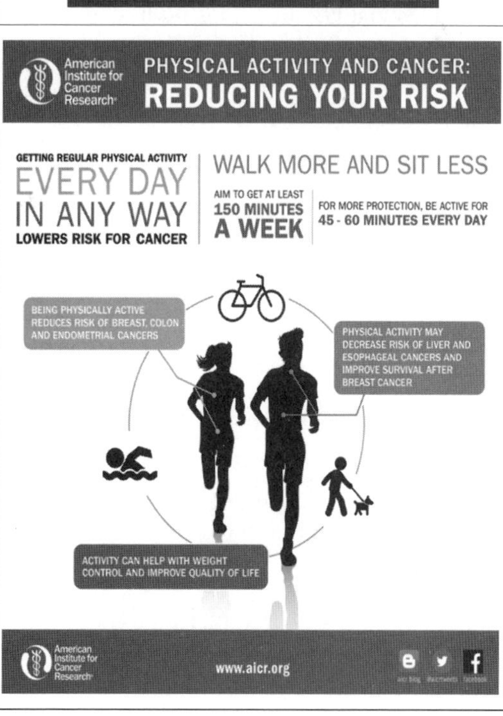

American Institute for Cancer Research
PHYSICAL ACTIVITY AND CANCER:
REDUCING YOUR RISK
GETTING REGULAR PHYSICAL ACTIVITY
EVERY DAY IN ANY WAY
LOWERS RISK FOR CANCER
WALK MORE AND SIT LESS
AIM TO GET AT LEAST 150 MINUTES A WEEK
FOR MORE PROTECTION, BE ACTIVE FOR 45 - 60 MINUTES EVERY DAY
BEING PHYSICALLY ACTIVE REDUCES RISK OF BREAST, COLON AND ENDOMETRIAL CANCERS
PHYSICAL ACTIVITY MAY DECREASE RISK OF LIVER AND ESOPHAGEAL CANCERS AND IMPROVE SURVIVAL AFTER BREAST CANCER
ACTIVITY CAN HELP WITH WEIGHT CONTROL AND IMPROVE QUALITY OF LIFE
American Institute for Cancer Research
www.aicr.org

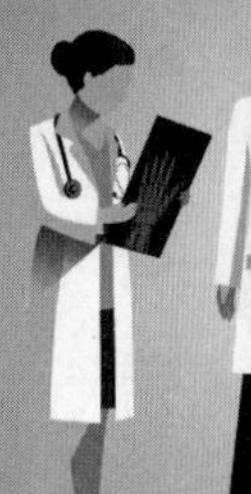

Physical Activity and Cancer
(ARGUMENT) Regular physical activity is one of the most important things people can do to improve their health…
(EVIDENCE) There is convincing evidence that…
(CONCLUSION) In general, the evidence implies that…

➢ To find more information about how to write with examples and statistics, you may refer to the following sources.

1. The Writing Center, University of Montana. 2020. Three ways to support an argument. Retrieved November 30, 2020, from the Writing Center, University of Montana website.
2. Fleming, G. 2020. Tips on how to write an argumentative essay. Retrieved November 27, 2020, from ThoughCo website.

Unit 7

Cancer

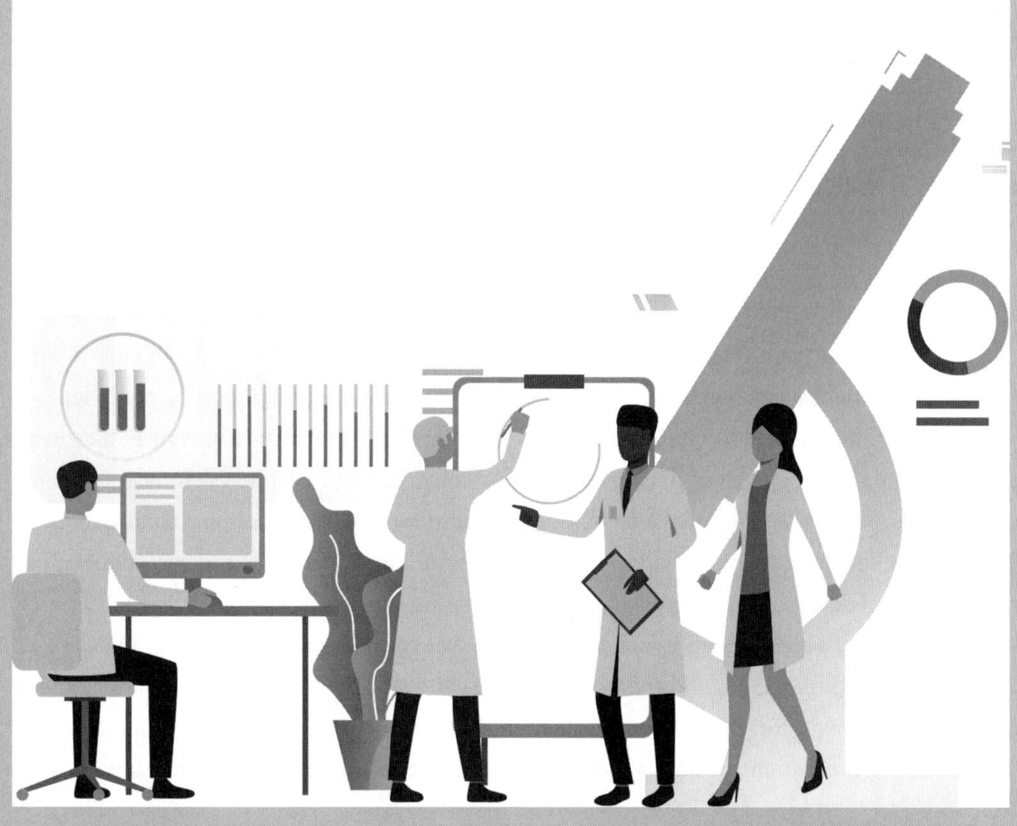

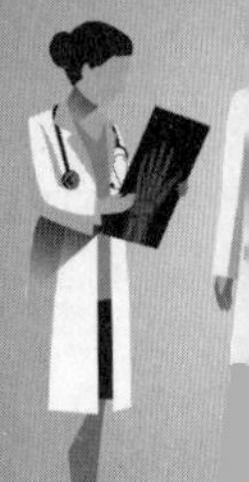

Part A | Information Searching and Delivering

I. Surf on the Internet and find information about the following topics before class.

1. chemotherapy
2. epidermal growth factor receptor (EGFR)
3. cervical cancer
4. breast carcinoma
5. non-small-cell lung cancer (NSCLC)

II. Make a presentation based on the information you've searched.

Part B | Text Understanding

Passage 1 Building a More Resilient Cancer Healthcare System

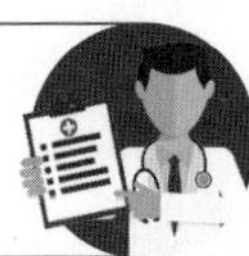

The outbreak of the COVID-19 pandemic has resulted in major disruptions to cancer care worldwide, including cancer screening programs. These interruptions will almost certainly lead to a surge in demand for cancer services that could overwhelm health systems. However, an increased focus on the prevention and early diagnosis of cancer could increase health-system resilience and lessen reliance on resource-intensive interventions, because early stage cancers can be treated more effectively and cost-efficiently than advanced stage disease. For this endeavor to succeed, clinical and technological developments in early cancer diagnosis are important.

With screening so important, it is a stark statistic that for lung cancer, screening rates are as low as 6% in at-risk populations compared with 60%–80% for breast, colon, or cervical cancer screening, even though early identification through screening can reduce the risk of lung cancer death by 20%. US research shows that nearly two-thirds of newly diagnosed patients with lung

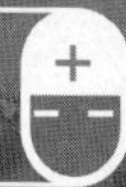

cancer do not meet the current US Preventive Services Task Force (USPSTF) criteria for annual lung cancer scans with low-dose CT, but have a similar risk of death to those who meet the criteria. In July, 2020, however, the USPSTF proposed updated recommendations that would nearly double the number of Americans currently offered annual scans by widening the eligibility criteria. The minimum age of inclusion would be reduced by 5 years to include adults aged 50–80 years who have a 20 pack-year smoking history, as opposed to the threshold of 30 pack-years in the current guidance. If approved, the new recommendations would also mean more women and more Black or African-American people would qualify for early screening.

Lung cancer is not a disease that is restricted to smokers. Around 10%–15% of patients with lung cancer in the UK have never smoked, while in East Asia, the incidence of lung cancer in non-smokers is about 53% and predominantly occurs in women. With non-smokers not necessarily meeting the criteria for lung cancer screening programs, understanding the early processes of lung carcinogenesis in non-smokers is necessary to ensure early detection. A study published in *Cell* in July, 2020, found that lung cancer in non-smokers is molecularly more diverse than lung cancer in smokers. Undertaking genomic, transcriptomic, proteomic, and phosphorylation analyses on 103 samples of early-stage non-small-cell lung cancer (NSCLC) tumors from non-smokers, Chen and colleagues found that tumors in women often had EGFR mutations whereas KRAS and APC gene alterations were more common in men. The study also found a high prevalence of APOBEC mutations in 75% of tumors from female patients younger than 60 years and genetic mutations resulting from exposure to environmental carcinogens, such as air pollution, in tumors from older women. These differences highlight not only a need for new treatments and diagnostic approaches for non-smokers with lung cancer, but also targeted interventions differentiated by sex.

On July 3, 2020, the UK Government together with various charities, announced a £16 million commitment to fund the development of integrated diagnostics to enable earlier detection and diagnosis of oesophageal, bowel, and lung cancer. As we move into the digital era, increased research into screening programs driven by artificial intelligence (AI) will provide major opportunities to aid earlier diagnosis. Indeed, many such research projects are underway. For example, data from the TRACERx study showed that AI-driven lung cancer screening combined with next-generation sequencing can map the evolution of lung cancer to predict clinical outcomes at the point of diagnosis. The study showed that patients with NSCLC who had less tumor immune activity were at an increased risk of relapse. Research such as this could transform the way cancer is diagnosed and better select those patients who are most likely to relapse and for whom treatments should be initiated earlier.

Building better resilience into cancer care systems is a clear lesson from COVID-19, and the pandemic provides an important opportunity to re-evaluate and re-configure strategies for global cancer control by directing available resources where they are most likely to have the largest benefit. All stakeholders should redouble their efforts on prevention and early detection to ensure

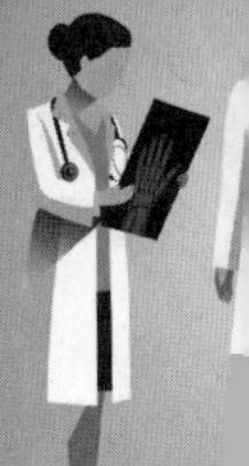

cancer healthcare systems are not stressed beyond breaking point in response to another highly disruptive event in the future.

Source: *The Lancet* Editorial Team. 2020. Building a more resilient cancer healthcare system. *The Lancet, 21*(8): 999.

I. Match the words with their definitions according to Passage 1.

____ 1. outbreak	ⓐ one of a system of tubes below the stomach in which solid waste collects before it is passed out of the body
____ 2. surge	ⓑ the level or point at which you start to experience sth., or at which sth. starts to happen
____ 3. stark	ⓒ to rearrange the elements or settings of (a system, device, computer application, etc.)
____ 4. scan	ⓓ to present sth. in detail
____ 5. threshold	ⓔ a promise to support sb./sth.
____ 6. target	ⓕ the sudden start of sth. unpleasant, especially violence or a disease
____ 7. commitment	ⓖ to get an image of an object, a part of sb.'s body, etc. on a computer by passing a beam of x-rays, ultrasound waves or electromagnetic waves over it in a special machine
____ 8. bowel	ⓗ clearly obvious to the eye or the mind
____ 9. map	ⓘ to try to have an effect on a particular group of people
____ 10. re-configure	ⓙ a sudden increase in the amount or number of sth.

II. Read Passage 1 and answer the following questions.

1. How can we build a more resilient cancer healthcare system according to the passage?

____

2. What lesson can we learn from COVID-19 according to the passage?

____

3. What benefit could the approval of the updated USPSTF recommendations bring about?

____

4. What do the findings of the study published in *Cell* in July, 2020 suggest?

____

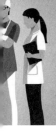

5. How does the author evaluate AI?

____

Passage 2 Disability in Cancer Care: Time for Change?

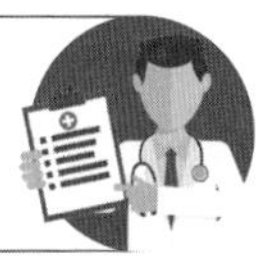

In the past few decades, numerous studies have found that the provision of timely cancer screening for individuals with physical disabilities is inadequate. Indeed, a report by the UK charity Jo's Cervical Cancer Trust, which surveyed 335 women with diverse physical disabilities and conditions, ranging from spinal muscular atrophy to cerebral palsy, found that a high proportion of respondents (63%) said that they had previously been unable to attend a cervical screening appointment because they could not access screening services or did not have the option for home visits. Moreover, nearly 40% stated that their general practice surgery did not provide wheelchair access, with just 1% of respondents reporting that their surgery provided a hoist. Approximately 13.9 million people in the UK are considered to have a disability, of whom 56% are women and most have impaired mobility. These findings are worrying in terms of equality of access to cancer care, especially in the context of global issues of overall health-care access for people with disabilities.

These findings are not confined to the UK. A study from the US in 2017 investigated how many people with and without disabilities received recommended breast, cervical, and colorectal cancer screening tests, stratified by disability type (hearing, vision, cognitive, and mobility). According to data from the 2013 National Health Interview Survey, individuals with disabilities, irrespective of type, reported fewer cancer screening test visits than those without disabilities, including pap tests, mammography, and colorectal cancer screening. The most frequent barriers to accessing screening services were difficulty in scheduling an appointment, long waiting times, and a lack of transportation to appointments. Although these barriers to access are common across many patient populations, these findings show that logistical difficulties can compound a situation in which people with disabilities are already disproportionally disadvantaged in terms of adequate health-care coverage. These disadvantages can include insurance cover (despite legal requirements to protect people with disabilities by the Americans with Disabilities Act), provider misperception about how to screen people with disabilities, insufficient experience with assistance for screening examinations, lack of equipment such as height-adjustable couches, geographical variation in the types of services offered, and lack of available outreach and education programs.

What both reports clearly show is that disparities persist among people with disabilities in need of preventive services and health-care access. Not only is increased awareness needed to identify gaps in accessing cancer screening services for those with disabilities, but also robust, comprehensive, and equitable interventions to ensure that such individuals are not overlooked for cancer screening. Moreover, incorrect assumptions are often made about people with disability—the result of common stigmas perpetuated by society—which include the inability to recognise long-term health conditions or debilitating symptoms that are not visible, or a belief that people with disabilities are not sexually active and therefore do not need health-care information about sexually transmitted infections, cervical cancer, or HIV. Given the diversity and complexity of disabilities that exist, it is imperative that healthcare practitioners recognise that individuals with disabilities are a heterogenous group with needs and requirements that will vary depending on the nature of their disabilities.

These prevailing issues can be addressed by some immediate and modest measures to increase the use of cancer care services for people with disabilities: increasing education in medical training on treating people with disability, both from a clinical perspective and regarding practical issues around medical procedures; improving accessibility to screening services in the primary-care setting; developing better education and outreach programs that specifically target people with disabilities; and ensuring fair and equal access to cancer services, regardless of geographical location. These policy interventions will be even more important given the existing shift from acute to chronic illnesses in high-income countries and their growing aging populations. Effective solutions are urgently needed to meet the health-care needs of individuals with disabilities and other vulnerable populations.

Source: *The Lancet* Editorial Team. 2019. Disability in cancer care: Time for change?. *The Lancet, 20*(9): 1183.

I. Match the words with their definitions according to Passage 2.

____ 1. provision	ⓐ to make sb.'s body or mind weaker
____ 2. respondent	ⓑ to arrange the different parts of something in separate layers or groups
____ 3. hoist	ⓒ consisting of many different kinds of people or things
____ 4. stratify	ⓓ to make worse by being an additional or intensifying factor
____ 5. mobility	ⓔ a person who answers questions, especially in a survey
____ 6. compound	ⓕ existing or most common at a particular time
____ 7. debilitate	ⓖ weak and easily hurt physically or emotionally
____ 8. heterogenous	ⓗ the act of supplying sb. with sth. that they need or want

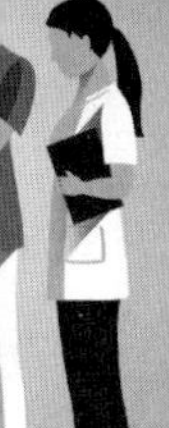

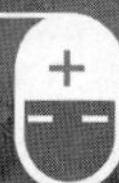

____ 9. prevailing	ⓘ	a piece of equipment used for lifting heavy things, or for lifting people who cannot stand or walk
____ 10. vulnerable	ⓙ	the ability to move or travel around easily

II. Read Passage 2 and answer the following questions.

1. What does the report by the UK charity Jo's Cervical Cancer Trust show?

____

2. In what aspects do people have difficulties in receiving cancer screening tests?

____

3. What should be done in order to improve the access of cancer screening services for people with disabilities?

____

4. What incorrect assumptions are held by the society toward people with physical disabilities?

____

5. What measures should be taken in order to improve the cancer care services for people with disabilities?

____

Passage 3 Time to Focus on Value-Based Metrics for Cancer Care?

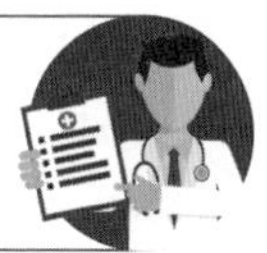

Despite dramatic advances in medicine, healthcare still causes harm too often, costs too much, and improves too slowly. This has led many payers and policy makers to focus on improving value, which includes quality, patient experience, and cost of care. Despite national attention on providing value in medicine, measures of value have been slow to emerge. We believe that professional societies have an opportunity to collaborate and develop standards that include not only outcomes but also patient experience and cost.

The breast program at our health system recently passed the National Accreditation Program for Breast Centers (NAPBC) re-accreditation process with no deficiencies. We are an American College of Radiology center of excellence and a National Cancer Institute—designated cancer center with Commission on Cancer accreditation. We routinely follow guidelines put forth by the

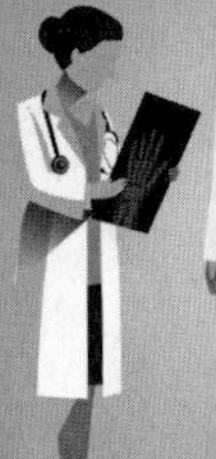

National Comprehensive Cancer Network, the American Society of Clinical Oncology, and the American Society for Radiation Oncology.

In the process of building a breast center of value and excellence, we developed a flow map of the patient's journey; what we encountered was humbling. Our time-to-treatment metrics were long, and our transitions of care were often chaotic. We realized that the designations and guidelines that we follow helped us provide one dimension of quality care—effective care, but did not always include other dimensions such as timely, patient-centered, and efficient care. We interviewed several patients as they went through their cancer treatment journey and found that "waiting" was a large component of their stress, as was worry about the financial burden. How could we be failing patients if we were passing our accreditations and following available guidelines?

There is an abundance of literature surrounding patient-centered care and value in medicine. The National Academy of Medicine developed a framework for advancing the quality of care, ensuring that care is safe, effective, efficient, patient-centered, timely, and equitable. Further work by the Picker Institute and Harvard explicated the domains of patient-centered care, the first of which is "respect for patient's values, preferences, and expressed needs." This information can help us focus on patients and improve value. Despite these frameworks, both the external accreditors and our internal care pathways missed several of these domains.

Patients have benefited greatly from guidelines in cancer care. These guidelines are generally organized, however, around the work of a specialty using evidence-based literature and expert consensus. The resulting recommendations focus on survival and recurrence but rarely include cost information, patient preferences, or "wait time suffering" as variables. These guidelines and standards are undoubtedly effective in improving the domain of quality. The NAPBC accreditation, for instance, requires the breast care team to undergo breast-specific continuing medical education, carry appropriate certification, and discuss their cases at multidisciplinary tumor boards. The NAPBC accreditation ensures that patients have access to components of cancer care such as genetics, irradiation, reconstruction, and survivorship. Finally, NAPBC accreditation mandates that programs follow national guidelines as part of their standard cancer treatment plan. While studies demonstrate that accreditation and the use of guidelines improve outcomes, we could do more to include other domains of quality such as ensuring care that is safe, efficient, patient-centered, and equitable. Guidelines that are oriented around all 6 National Academy of Medicine domains of quality and encompass the entire continuum of care offer hope to improve the value of care delivered.

For patients with cancer, delays in treatment lead to a worse prognosis. Recent studies evaluating time to first treatment suggest that for every week delay in diagnosis or treatment,

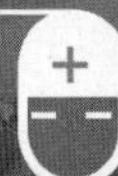

mortality is increased by more than 1%. Yet due to increasing complexities in treatment, access issues, and delays from insurance approvals, the time to treatment is getting longer instead of shorter. For patients with cancer, time waiting for a diagnosis or treatment is suffering. What are reasonable metrics for "waiting" that are focused on patient suffering in addition to survival? Expanding current guidelines to include time-based measures between points of care will improve not only outcomes but patient satisfaction. We have an opportunity to work with patients and various societies to delineate ideal wait times for treatments and transitions of care based on outcomes data and patient anxiety.

Cancer care can also be improved by incorporating cost information into performance measures. There is evidence that in the US, we overtreat many patients with cancer who then pay for a treatment (financially and with adverse effects) that has very little benefit. Cost savings will result from decreasing treatment variation, improving efficiency, and assessing efficacy by personalizing care. Examples of this include using genomic testing to determine who can avoid chemotherapy, following guidelines to identify patients in whom intraoperative irradiation could spare weeks of external-beam therapy, and providing services in patient's homes rather than hospitals. Standards are available for each component of the patient's care based on survival and recurrence. We also need to improve the transitions between touch points of care in the patient's treatment journey to reduce the anxiety associated with waiting. Financial implications, adverse effects, and patient preferences could be incorporated into recommendations along with information on alternative therapies. Shared decision-making needs to be a component of our standards. Finally, we need to address and eliminate inequities in care.

Health care is migrating from a fee-for-service model to a value-based or shared-risk model of reimbursement; our metrics and incentives should also be value based. It is time for standards of cancer care to include patient experience and cost in addition to traditional quality metrics. Societies that have a stake in breast cancer care have an opportunity to partner with each other and with patients to create holistic value-based guidelines that, if embraced, will further improve cancer care. The American College of Surgeons' quality and cancer programs are currently developing value-based metrics. The NAPBC has representation from all disciplines, including patient advocacy groups, and is well suited to lead this effort. There is no need to wait for a cure for many patients with breast cancer at our institutions. We have the cure if we work together with those we serve.

Source: Dietz, J. R & Pronovost, P. 2020. Time to Focus on Value-Based Metrics for Cancer Care?. *JAMA Oncology, 6*(9): 1325-1326.

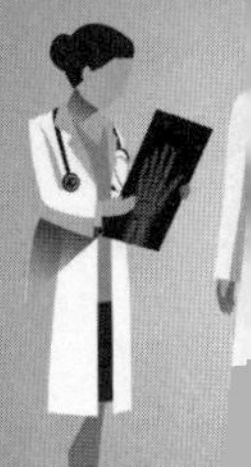

I. Match the words with their definitions according to Passage 3.

____ 1. designation	ⓐ uninterrupted existence or succession
____ 2. irradiation	ⓑ compensation paid (to someone) for damages or losses or money already spent etc.
____ 3. orient	ⓒ the giving of public support to an idea, a course of action or a belief
____ 4. mandate	ⓓ to shift, as from one system or enterprise to another
____ 5. continuum	ⓔ to describe, draw or explain sth. in detail
____ 6. delineate	ⓕ to direct sb./sth. towards sth.
____ 7. alternative	ⓖ to order sb. to behave, do sth. or vote in a particular way
____ 8. migrate	ⓗ name, description, or title, typically one that is officially bestowed
____ 9. reimbursement	ⓘ different from the usual or traditional way in which sth. is done
____ 10. advocacy	ⓙ the therapeutic or diagnostic use of radiation, esp. x-rays

II. Read Passage 3 and answer the following questions.

1. What do value-based metrics of cancer care refer to according to the passage?

   ____

2. What is the author's opinion on the current guidelines in the passage?

   ____

3. What could be the possible results of delays in treatment?

   ____

4. How to improve the value of cancer care?

   ____

5. What is the trend of cancer care in the future according to the passage?

   ____

III. Read the three passages comprehensively and answer the following questions.

1. What is the common theme of the three passages?

   ____

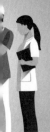

2. What is the main writing skill of Passage 1 and Passage 2?

____

3. In your opinion, how to improve cancer care in our country?

____

4. Write a short passage of about 100 words to synthesize the information of the three passages.

____

____

____

____

____

Part C Integrated Exercises

I. Read the words below, and pay attention to the pronunciation. Use the scale below (1, 2, 3) to give yourself a score for each word. Try to consult your dictionary for the words with score 1.

❶ I don't understand this word.
❷ I understand this word when I see it or hear it, but I don't know how to use it.
❸ I know this word and can use it in my own speaking and writing.

Academic words

□ accreditation	□ adverse	□ advocacy	□ alteration
□ chaotic	□ collaborate	□ continuum	□ coverage
□ debilitate	□ delineate	□ designation	□ differentiate
□ disparity	□ disproportionally	□ disruptive	□ dramatic
□ drive	□ eligibility	□ eliminate	□ endeavor
□ explicate	□ fund	□ heterogenous	□ holistic
□ humbling	□ impaired	□ incorporate	□ initiate
□ logistical	□ mandate	□ map	□ metric
□ migrate	□ misperception	□ mobility	□ orient
□ outbreak	□ outreach	□ overlook	□ perpetuate
□ propose	□ provision	□ qualify	□ re-configure

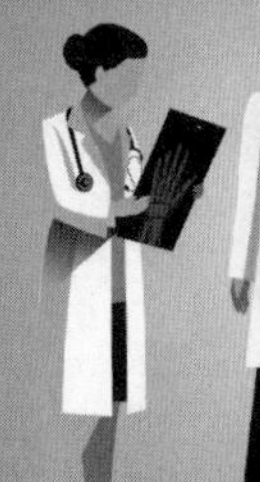

- □ recommend
- □ reimbursement
- □ restrict
- □ robust
- □ sequencing
- □ stark
- □ state
- □ stigma
- □ stratify
- □ surge
- □ target
- □ undertake
- □ urgently
- □ widen

Discipline-specific words

- □ atrophy
- □ bowel
- □ carcinogenesis
- □ cerebral
- □ cervical
- □ chemotherapy
- □ colon
- □ colorectal
- □ disability
- □ dose
- □ genetic
- □ genomic
- □ hoist
- □ immune
- □ intervention
- □ intraoperative
- □ irradiation
- □ mammography
- □ molecularly
- □ muscular
- □ mutation
- □ oncology
- □ overtreat
- □ palsy
- □ patient-centered
- □ phosphorylation
- □ proteomic
- □ radiology
- □ reconstruction
- □ relapse
- □ sample
- □ scan
- □ spinal
- □ surgery
- □ survivorship
- □ transcriptomic
- □ tumor
- □ vulnerable

II. Match each word in the box with the group of words that regularly occur in academic writing.

perpetuate	overlook	recommend	state	eliminate
propose	widen	restrict	undertake	fund

1. ______________ a toast / a method / a bill
2. ______________ one's knowledge / the gap / inequality
3. ______________ a mission / responsibility / a role
4. ______________ discrimination / poverty / waste
5. ______________ a fact / one's reason / one's belief
6. ______________ a product / a surgery / a route
7. ______________ the memory / a tradition / the myth
8. ______________ a fault / a flaw / a small detail
9. ______________ one's freedom / one's rights / the speed
10. ______________ the education / a school / a campaign

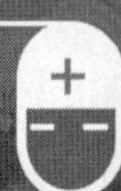

III. Study the members of the word families in the table below. Try to work out the meaning in each case according to its prefix or suffix.

The members of a word family	Chinese definitions
disrupt, disruptive, disruption	使瓦解、分裂的、瓦解
rely, reliable, reliance, unreliable	
alter, alterable, alterability, alteration	
differ, difference, differential, differentiate	
gene, genetic, genome, genomic	
carcinogen, carcinogenic, carcinogenesis	
esophagus, esophageal, esophagectomy	
oncology, oncological, oncologist	
accredit, accreditor, accreditation	
survive, survival, survivor, survivorship	
recur, recurrent, recurrence	
construct, reconstruct, reconstruction	
proportion, proportional, disproportional, disproportionally	
disable, disabled, disability	
mammography, mammogram, mammoplasty	
muscle, muscular, muscularity	
atrophy, dystrophy, hypotrophy, hypertrophy	
sex, sexual, sexually	
cerebrum, cerebral, cerebrovascular	
prevent, preventive, prevention	

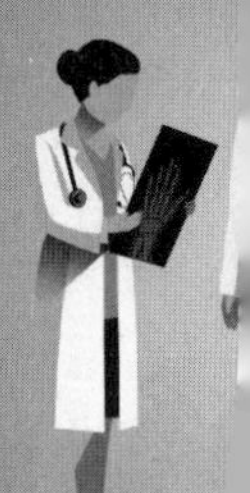

IV. Complete each sentence below with a word from the table above.

1. Dozens of patients had their operations postponed because of the ________ operating tables. (rely)
2. This ________ is thought to be mostly the result of the immune response to the virus. (alter)
3. Recent reports suggest that adult stem cells can ________ into developmentally unrelated cell types. (differ)
4. Establishment of an early and reliable biomarker for oral ________ will enable early diagnosis of cancer. (carcinogen)
5. She had even been referred by the ________ for an experimental trial of chemotherapy. (oncology)
6. It provides a forum for sharing essential, evidence-based information and perspectives on progress in cancer research, ________ and advocacy. (survive)
7. The disorder is thus characterised by involuntary, persistent remembering or reliving the traumatic event in flashbacks, vivid memories, and ________ dreams. (recur)
8. The morbidity and mortality of the host species are usually ________ to the number of coccidial oocysts ingested. (proportion)
9. Yoga has been proven to aid the development of self-esteem in severely ________ children. (disable)
10. Hearty laughter increases heart rate, blood pressure and respiratory rate, and ________ activity. (muscle)

V. Choose the word in each list that is not a synonym for the underlined word.

1. <u>dramatic</u>
   A. impressive B. exciting C. striking D. ordinary
2. <u>collaborate</u>
   A. cooperate B. compete C. ally D. associate
3. <u>chaotic</u>
   A. orderly B. disorganized C. messy D. confused
4. <u>explicate</u>
   A. explain B. bewilder C. expound D. clarify
5. <u>holistic</u>
   A. whole B. comprehensive C. fragmentary D. integrated

6. impaired
   A. damaged B. disabled C. intact D. afflicted
7. robust
   A. strong B. weak C. tough D. powerful
8. approximately
   A. exactly B. roughly C. nearly D. almost
9. abundance
   A. plenty B. mass C. profusion D. scarcity
10. equitable
   A. impartial B. biased C. fair D. just

VI. Read the following expressions and sentence patterns aloud and analyze the formality of the structures used.

Target sentence patterns

1. **With** screening so important, it is a stark statistic that for lung cancer, screening rates are **as low as** 6% in at-risk populations **compared with** 60%–80% for breast, colon, or cervical cancer screening, **even though** early identification through screening can reduce the risk of lung cancer death by 20%.
2. The minimum age of inclusion would be reduced by 5 years to include adults aged 50–80 years who have a 20 pack-year smoking history, **as opposed to** the threshold of 30 pack-years in the current guidance.
3. Chen and colleagues found that tumors in women often had EGFR mutations **whereas** KRAS and APC gene alterations were **more common in** men.
4. Data from the TRACERx study showed that AI-driven lung cancer screening **combined with** next-generation sequencing can map the evolution of lung cancer to predict clinical outcomes **at the point of** diagnosis.
5. The study showed that patients with NSCLC who had less tumor immune activity were **at** an increased **risk of** relapse.
6. Building better resilience into cancer care systems is **a** clear **lesson from** COVID-19.
7. All stakeholders should redouble their efforts on prevention and early detection to ensure cancer healthcare systems are not stressed beyond breaking point **in response to** another highly disruptive event in the future.

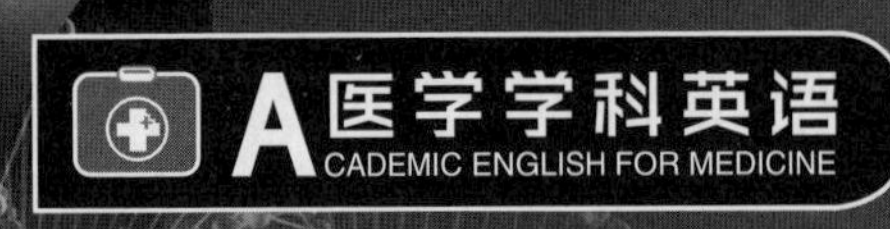

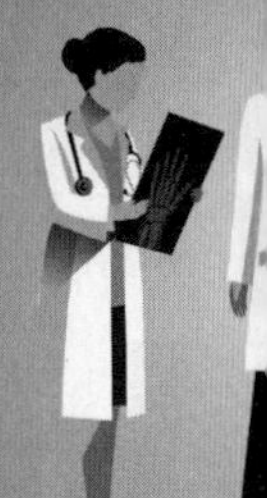

8. We routinely follow guidelines **put forth by** the National Comprehensive Cancer Network, the American Society of Clinical Oncology, and the American Society for Radiation Oncology.
9. We interviewed several patients as they **went through** their cancer treatment journey and found that "waiting" was a large component of their stress, as was worry about the financial burden.
10. There is **an abundance of** literature surrounding patient-centered care and value in medicine.
11. Patients have **benefited greatly from** guidelines in cancer care.
12. What are reasonable metrics for "waiting" that **are focused on** patient suffering **in addition to** survival?
13. Cost savings will **result from** decreasing treatment variation, improving efficiency, and assessing efficacy by personalizing care.
14. Standards **are available for** each component of the patient's care **based on** survival and recurrence.
15. Health care is **migrating from** a fee-for-service model to a value-based or shared-risk model of reimbursement; our metrics and incentives should also be value based.
16. **It is time for** standards of cancer care **to** include patient experience and cost in addition to traditional quality metrics.
17. Financial implications, adverse effects, and patient preferences could **be incorporated into** recommendations **along with** information on alternative therapies.
18. Societies that **have a stake in** breast cancer care have an opportunity to partner with each other and with patients to create holistic value-based guidelines that, if embraced, will further improve cancer care.
19. The NAPBC has representation from all disciplines, including patient advocacy groups, and **is well suited to** lead this effort.
20. **Indeed**, a report by the UK charity Jo's Cervical Cancer Trust, which surveyed 335 women with diverse physical disabilities and conditions, **ranging from** spinal muscular atrophy **to** cerebral palsy, found that **a high proportion of** respondents (63%) said that they had previously been unable to attend a cervical screening appointment because they could not access screening services or did not **have the option for** home visits.
21. These findings are worrying **in terms of** equality of access to cancer care, especially **in the context of** global issues of overall health-care access for people with disabilities.
22. These findings **are** not **confined to** the UK. A study from the US in 2017 investigated how many people with and without disabilities received recommended breast, cervical, and colorectal cancer screening tests, stratified by disability type (hearing, vision, cognitive, and mobility).
23. **According to** data from the 2013 National Health Interview Survey, individuals with disabilities, **irrespective of** type, reported fewer cancer screening test visits than those without

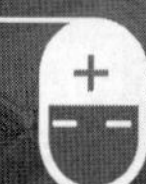

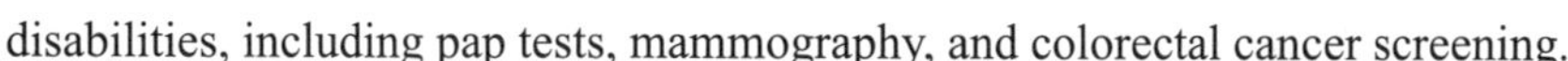

disabilities, including pap tests, mammography, and colorectal cancer screening.

24. **Given** the diversity and complexity of disabilities that exist, **it is imperative that** healthcare practitioners recognise that individuals with disabilities are a heterogenous group with needs and requirements that will vary **depending on** the nature of their disabilities.
25. Effective solutions are urgently needed to **meet the** health-care **needs** of individuals with disabilities and other vulnerable populations

VII. For each of the sentences below, write a new sentence as similar as possible in meaning to the original one, but as formal as possible in style.

1. He is likely to accept this therapy, which is different from the previous one.

2. This law against abortion is suggested by the first female super court judge.

3. Why is there a lot of thymine base in the neighborhood of breast cancer mutations?

4. Proteins are used in the construction of each cell of every organ, gland or system as well as the muscular structure.

5. Normally, inflammation occurs when white blood cells move from the blood, through the blood vessel wall and into the surrounding tissue.

6. All the countries have much to do with preventing sudden and catastrophic infectious diseases.

7. Because the drug is affordable and does not require cold storage, it fits resource-poor settings very well.

8. The heart muscle of the strength athletes, however, tended to thicken, a phenomenon that appeared to be limited to the left ventricle.

9. Acidosis can occur in spite of the amount of oxygen in the air being breathed.

10. Because of these findings, we must note that adequate iron is provided in infancy and early childhood.

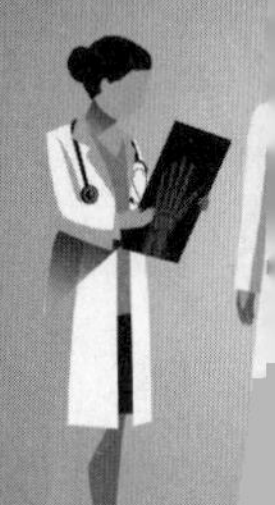

VIII. Translate the following sentences by using the following words and phrases. Make sure that your English sentences are different from the Chinese versions in terms of structures or orders, but as formal as possible. Then compare yours with your partner's according to the criteria: Whose version is more different and more formal?

1. 新的研究表明，个子高的人患癌症的风险更高，因为他们体内的细胞更多。(at a risk of)

____

2. 晚期前列腺癌的治疗反应存在种族差异。(in response to)

____

3. 过去的经验教训是，高血压是中风最重要的可改变的危险因素。(a lesson from)

____

4. 如果是那样的话，我们就必须对这些女性积极进行随访，确保她们通过治疗受益。(benefit from)

____

5. 他说他们来北京是因为他的妻子要做一个胃部手术。(go through)

____

6. 预防工作是奏效的，但必须把重点放在那些最有可能接触艾滋病毒的人群上，同时也必须具有持续性。(be focused on)

____

7. 现在是世界各国联合起来对付这种传染病的时候了。(it is time for...to)

____

8. 怀孕的病人有权选择在分娩时将她们的脐带血采集和储存以供将来使用。(have the option for)

____

9. 研究人员特别针对儿童的神经发育情况进行跟踪评估。(in terms of)

____

10. 该系统图像清晰，性能稳定，能够满足医疗检测的需要。(meet the need of)

____

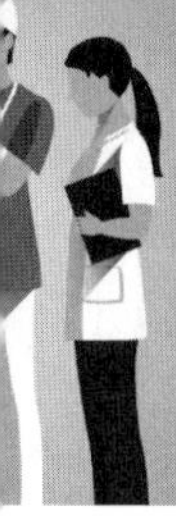

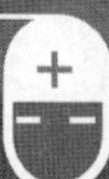

Part D | Academic Skills

Academic Listening Skill

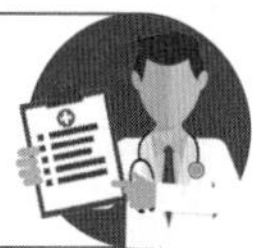

Recognizing Cause and Effect Relationship

Recognizing cause and effect is a common method of organizing ideas when listening. Identifying cause and effect involves understanding how come things happen (cause) and what happens as a result (effect). When you figure out why something happens and what happens as a result, this will help you understand better what a speaker is talking about and the logic of the listening material. Here are some expressions that indicate cause and effect relationship: so, since, as a result, hence, thereby, etc. In order to comprehend the passage, we need to take some notes. Efficient notetakers do not write down every word for a lecture, they can use abbreviations for common words or for a specific word. There are many ways to abbreviate. Figure out what abbreviations make sense to you. Here are some examples:

1. shorten long words to one or two syllables, such as genetics = gene;
2. leave out the vowels, such as mutation = mution;
3. use a single letter for a high-frequency word, such as cancer = c

Listening 1

Word bank

1. RNA	abbreviation for ribonucleic acid, which is an important chemical present in all living cells
2. molecule	the simplest unit of a chemical substance, usually a group of two or more atoms

3. mitosis	the type of cell division in which one cell divides into two cells that are exactly the same, each with the same number of chromosomes as the original cell
4. mutation	the way in which genes change and produce permanent differences
5. mechanism	a way of doing something that is planned or part of a system
6. carcinogen	a substance that can cause cancer
7. offspring	a person's children
8. non-communicable	cannot be passed from one person to another

I. Listen to the passage and choose the best answer to each of the questions.

❶ What does the passage mainly talk about?

Ⓐ Cancer starts when cells begin to grow and multiply too much.

Ⓑ Lifestyle is one of the many factors which will trigger cancer.

Ⓒ Cancer is the result of changes in cells that lead to uncontrolled self-growth and division.

Ⓓ There is no doubt that a normal cell turns into a cancer cell when too many proteins are produced.

❷ Which of the following options cannot trigger cancer?

Ⓐ Smoking.

Ⓑ Genetics.

Ⓒ UV radiation.

Ⓓ Unhealthy eating habits.

II. Listen to the passage and fill in the blanks by taking notes.

What can cause mutations?	**1.** Mutations can happen by ________.
	2. Mutations can also be triggered by ________.
	3. ________ also have a role to play.
	4. Other factors include ____.

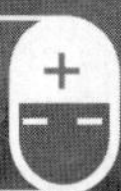

III. Listen to the passage and decide whether the following statements are true (T) or false (F).

________ 1. Proteins and RNA together control the cell.
________ 2. Human body is made up of between 50 and 75 trillion cells.
________ 3. Cancer is a non-communicable disease among humans.
________ 4. Primary tumors can start at a fixed place in people's body.
________ 5. The life span of white blood cells is on average over two years.

IV. Write down the abbreviations of words from the passage in your own way according to the above rules of abbreviation.

1. protein ________
2. radiation ________
3. abnormal ________
4. cell ________
5. carcinogen ________

Listening 2

Word bank

1. harness	to control and use the force or strength of sth. to produce power or to achieve sth.
2. eradicate	to destroy or get rid of sth. completely, especially sth. bad
3. pox	any disease characterized by the formation of pustules on the skin that often leave pockmarks when healed
4. metastasize	to spread throughout the body
5. chemotherapy	the treatment of disease, especially cancer, with the use of chemical substances
6. immunotherapy	the treatment or prevention of disease by taking measures to increase immune system functioning

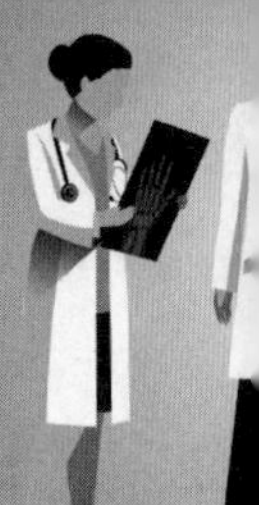

7. culture	(1) a group of cells or bacteria, especially one taken from a person or an animal and grown for medical or scientific study, or to produce food (2) to grow a group of cells or bacteria for medical or scientific study
8. subclone	a clone or descendant of a mutant occurring in a previous clone
9. glioblastoma	a fast-growing malignant brain tumor composed of spongioblasts
10. heterogeneity	the quality or state of consisting of dissimilar or diverse elements
11. vanquish	to defeat sb. completely in a competition, war, etc.
12. residual	remaining at the end of a process
13. bombard	to attack a place by firing large guns at it or dropping bombs on it continuously
14. mortality	the number of deaths in a particular situation or period of time
15. arsenal	a building where military weapons and explosives are made or stored

I. Listen to the passage and choose the best answer to each of the questions.

❶ **Why is it so hard to cure cancer according to the passage?**

Ⓐ It is because some cancers are malignant.

Ⓑ It is because the treatments are so damaging. Sometimes the patients die before the cancer is cured.

Ⓒ It is because treating cancer is too expensive for many people.

Ⓓ It is because cancer is incredibly complex. There are more than 100 different types and we don't have a magic bullet that can cure all of them.

❷ **Which of the following statements is NOT true?**

Ⓐ Existing treatments are very far from 100% effective.

Ⓑ Clonal heterogeneity makes treatment difficult.

Ⓒ Figuring out how to target stubborn cells will surely prevent cancers from coming back.

Ⓓ Cancer cells are adjusting their molecular and cellular characteristics to survive under stress.

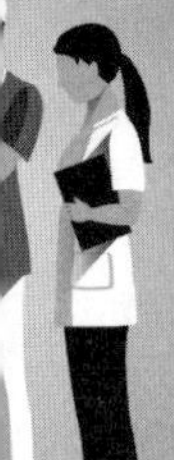

Unit 7 Cancer

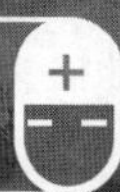

II. Listen to the passage again and answer the following questions.

1. What causes cancer according to the passage?

   ____

2. What are the effective treatments for cancer in many cases according to the passage?

   1) Treatments usually include a combination of ____________________ and ____________________ and ____________________ to kill any cancerous cells left behind.

   2) ____________________, ____________________, and ____________________ tailored for a specific type of cancers are sometimes used too.

III. Listen to the passage again and match the methods 1-4 with the causes A-D.

________ 1. We need new, better ways of studying cancer.

________ 2. We should learn how to shut down the cancer cells' communication in the dynamic interconnected ecosystem.

________ 3. We need to figure out how to eradicate cancer stem cells.

________ 4. We need to find experimental systems that match cancers' complexity, and monitoring and treatment options that can adjust as the cancer changes.

Ⓐ It is because cancer cells can induce normal cells to form blood vessels that feed the tumor and remove waste products. And they can also interact with the immune system to actually suppress its function, keeping it from recognizing or destroying the cancer.

Ⓑ It is because these cells can make them resistant to chemotherapy and radiation.

Ⓒ It is because some cancer cells can effectively switch on protective shields against whatever's attacking them by changing their gene expression. Malignant cancers are complex systems that constantly evolve and adapt.

Ⓓ It is because cultured cells lack much of the complexity of a tumor in an actual living organism.

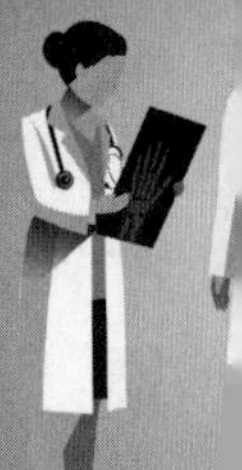

Academic Reading Skill

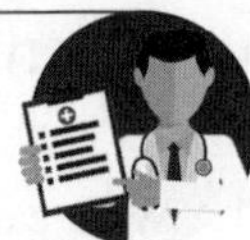

Arguments and Evidences

Argument is an essential part of academic writing. Making arguments is expressing our points of view, the reasoning of which requires employing a series of relevant evidences. Therefore, we use evidences to support our reasons, and all the reasons together make our claim convincing. We can see evidences are indispensable in argument writing in that they support the veracity of the claims made by us. Actually, evidences in argument writing are often acquired from another people's work. To incorporate their works into our claims requires three methods: *quoting, paraphrasing*, and *summarizing*.

There are four types of evidence the author can use to make claims reasonable, namely *anecdotes, facts, quotes* and *statistics.* Anecdotes derive from personal or other's experiences. Using examples helps provide specific details and add vividness to the argument. Facts are indisputable, which makes it a powerful means of convincing. Citing quotes from leading authorities and experts is a useful logical appeal to support the claims we make. Though it serves as an interpretation of the facts, it is widely accepted in academic writing to back up the arguments. Meanwhile, it is an essential ethical principle to mention the source of the quotes. Statistics is also referred to as data. It is regarded as an excellent and convincing means since it represents facts and logic. It is worth mentioning that evidences are not limited to the four types. Besides, they vary with disciplines. In some hard science like engineering, data are frequently used evidences. But in soft science, like history, literature may be used as evidences.

No matter what type of evidence is used in the claims, we should always keep in mind that the evidences we select should be *relevant, typical, accurate*, and *sufficient* to the claims. Relevance means the evidences should be pertinent to the arguments and support the claims. Being typical and representative suggests that the evidences should neither be aberrant nor one-sided, and rather, it should cover a full range of opinions and represent typical opinions of the experts or authorities. Accuracy means that the data used should be accurate. To guarantee accuracy requires using up-to-date data instead of using out-of-date data, or it would lower the credibility of the author. At last, being sufficient means that we should provide enough evidences to support our claims.

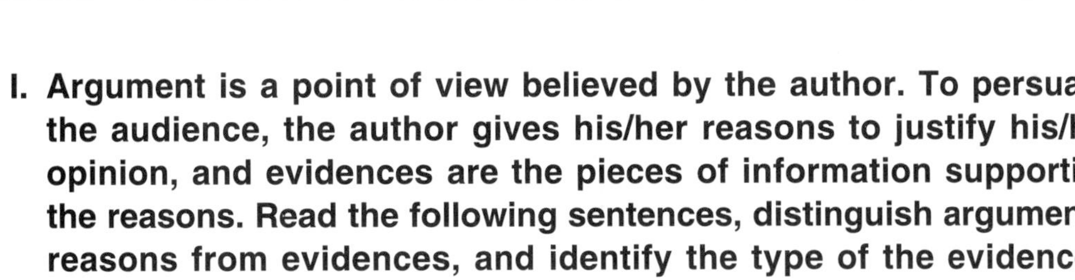

Unit 7 Cancer

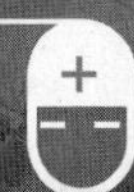

I. Argument is a point of view believed by the author. To persuade the audience, the author gives his/her reasons to justify his/her opinion, and evidences are the pieces of information supporting the reasons. Read the following sentences, distinguish arguments, reasons from evidences, and identify the type of the evidences. Then fill in the blanks below.

❶ ① Clinical and technological developments in early cancer diagnosis are important. ② In July, 2020, however, the USPSTF proposed updated recommendations that would nearly double the number of Americans currently offered annual scans by widening the eligibility criteria. ③ The minimum age of inclusion would be reduced by 5 years to include adults aged 50–80 years who have a 20 pack-year smoking history, as opposed to the threshold of 30 pack-years in the current guidance. ④ If approved, the new recommendations would also mean more women and more Black or African-American people would qualify for early screening.

❷ ① There is an abundance of literature surrounding patient-centered care and value in medicine. ② The National Academy of Medicine developed a framework for advancing the quality of care, ensuring that care is safe, effective, efficient, patient centered, timely, and equitable. ③ Further work by the Picker Institute and Harvard explicated the domains of patient-centered care, the first of which is "respect for patient's values, preferences, and expressed needs."

❸ ① Cancer care can also be improved by incorporating cost information into performance measures. ② There is evidence that in the US, we overtreat many patients with cancer who then pay for a treatment (financially and with adverse effects) that has very little benefit. ③ Cost savings will result from decreasing treatment variation, improving efficiency, and assessing efficacy by personalizing care. ④ Examples of this include using genomic testing to determine who can avoid chemotherapy, following guidelines to identify patients in whom intraoperative irradiation could spare weeks of external-beam therapy, and providing services in patient's homes rather than hospitals.

❹ ① Teamwork matters in all healthcare, but it really impacts cancer treatments. ② "Advancing cancer care requires more than just science. It's a collective effort driven by passionate individuals and organizations dedicated to making a difference for those living with and affected by cancer," says Olivier Nataf, head of US Oncology at AstraZeneca. ③ "There is tremendous work being done across the cancer community today, and we have a responsibility to amplify efforts from those making change in cancer care and finding ways to bring groups together."

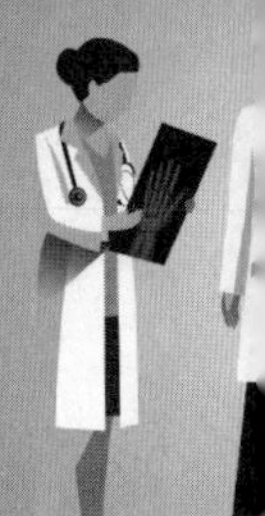

No.	Arguments	Reasons	Evidences			
			Anecdotal Evidence	Factual Evidence	Quote Evidence	Statistical Evidence
1						
2						
3						
4						

II. Match each argument in column A with the evidence in column B. Make sure that your choice follows the principle of relevance.

Column A (argument)	Column B (evidence)
1. Good communication between patients, family caregivers, and the health care team is very important in cancer care.	A. In the US, bladder cancer is expected to strike about 53,000 men and 18,000 women this year.
2. AI has significant potential to cope with some of these burning healthcare problems, including cancer.	B. "A couple of years ago the big story was that immunotherapy can work," Jedd Wolchok, director of immunotherapy at the Ludwig Center at Memorial Sloan-Kettering Cancer Center told Bloomberg. "Now immunotherapy has entered the mainstream."
3. Cancer immunotherapy is important.	C. Studies show that when patients and doctors communicate well during cancer care, there are many positive results. Patients are usually more satisfied with the care and feel more in control, and more likely to follow through with treatment.
4. Gender affects one's cancer risks.	D. Take the example of oncology, which is one of the areas we are specifically focusing on. There are 70,000 new studies, articles and pieces of evidence every year in oncology. This cannot be tapped into by an individual. However, IBM can feign a system to assist with orientation and bring forward the relevant pieces of the information.

➢ To find more information about evidence-based essays, you may refer to the following sources.

1. Robin, J. 2023. Types of evidence in academic arguments. Retrieved April 8, 2023, from Pressbooks website.
2. Emilie, Z. 2023. Failures in evidence: When even "lots of quotes" can't save an argument. Retrieved April 8, 2023, from Pressbooks website.
3. The Writing Center, University of North Carolina at Chapel Hill. 2020. Evidence. Retrieved August 30, 2020, from the Writing Center, University of North Carolina at Chapel Hill website.

Academic Writing Skill

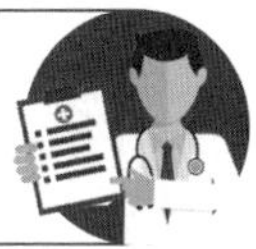

Quoting and Paraphrasing

To provide evidence to support your argument and avoid plagiarism, you need to incorporate other writers' work into your own writing, so you need to master the literacy skill of citation. According to the closeness of your writing to the source writing, there are three methods of citation: quoting, paraphrasing and summarizing. This unit focuses on the first two kinds.

Being the most convenient way, **quoting** refers to copying the exact words from the original source and placing quotation marks around the words. There are several ways to integrate quotations into your text. Often, a short quotation works well when integrated into a sentence, for example: *During the 1970s, the US began what has now become known as the "war on drugs," a reaction to the counterculture and drug-fueled climate of the 1960s.* Longer quotations can stand alone, for example: *Kidder noted that "providing sick people with medicine, but no food, is like washing one's hands and drying them off in the dirt."* However, quotations should not be overused in your writing, and whenever possible it is preferable to use your own words to interpret other sources with paraphrasing and summarizing.

Paraphrasing involves rewriting the words in your own words to make them different to the source yet retain all the meaning, for example: (Original) *Symptoms of the flu include fever and nasal congestion.*→(Paraphrase) *Stuffiness and elevated temperature are signs of the flu.* Paraphrased material is usually slightly shorter than the original passage.

Obviously, paraphrasing is more difficult than direct quoting, but there are some tips. You can paraphrase the sentences by using synonyms (e.g. change "show" to "demonstrate"), by changing the verb form (e.g. from active to passive), by changing the word class (e.g. from verb to noun), or

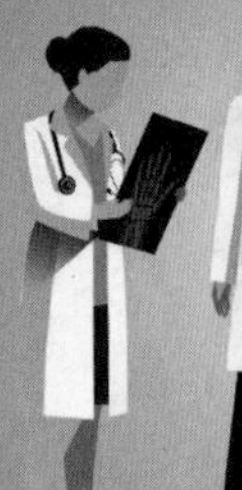

by using different forms of sentence structure (e.g. break the information into separate sentences).

No matter which kind you adopt, the original source should be acknowledged. As follows, there are mainly three versions of citation.

1) **Information-focused**

Give priority to the information over the author(s) with the citation at the end of the sentence.

➢ *Tuberculosis is a disease that is more commonly found in individuals living in poverty, and it is also a cause of extreme socioeconomic stress. (Reid et al., 2019)*

2) **Author-focused**

Place the author(s)'s name(s) in the subject position in the sentence.

➢ *Sudfeld and colleagues (2020) found that although vitamin D3 was well tolerated, there was no effect of vitamin D3 supplementation on the risk of mortality.*

3) **Weak author-focused**

Use "researchers" or "statisticians" or other identities instead of the names of the authors in the sentence.

➢ *Researchers indicate that increased levels of carbon dioxide in the atmosphere are reducing levels of nutrients (such as zinc, iron, calcium, and potassium) in wheat, barley, potatoes, and rice. (Myers et al., 2014)*

In addition, the following **reporting verbs** and **structures** are commonly used while quoting and paraphrasing.

As sb. / Sb. / The research by sb.	shows / observes / points out / remarks / says / states / argues / claims / concludes / suggests / notes	that... / that "...".

- To quote sb. "..."
- According to sb..../ "..."
- As noted by sb..../ "..."
- In sb.'s view.../ "..."

I. Identify the citation methods and citation versions used in the given citations.

Citations	Citation methods	Citation versions
1. The National Academy of Medicine developed a framework for advancing the quality of care, ensuring that care is safe, effective, efficient, patient centered, timely, and equitable.		

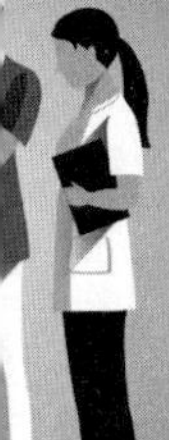

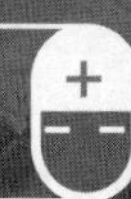

2. Further work by the Picker Institute and Harvard explicated the domains of patient-centered care, the first of which is "respect for patient's values, preferences, and expressed needs."		
3. When mucus hardens, it becomes more difficult to cough which is our way of trying to expel mucus and the germs it contains (Schaffner, 2014).		
4. Recent studies evaluating time to first treatment suggest that for every week delay in diagnosis or treatment, mortality is increased by more than 1%.		

II. Paraphrase the following sentences based on the mentioned tips.

1. "You have to make yourself drink fluids, even though all you want to do is collapse," says William Schaffner.

   ____

   ____

2. Overweight and obesity is associated with increased total mortality and increased risk of cardiovascular diseases, diabetes, and several types of cancer. It does so by increasing high blood pressure, blood cholesterol, insulin resistance and inflammation.

   ____

   ____

   ____

   ____

3. Although white rice accounts for 35%-80% of the caloric intake for 3.3 billion Asians, it has several problems, such as lack of adequate nutrition, which makes Asian's body size relatively small; and also a lack of taste, which leads to high consumption of sodium in many of the foods eaten with rice.

   ____

   ____

   ____

   ____

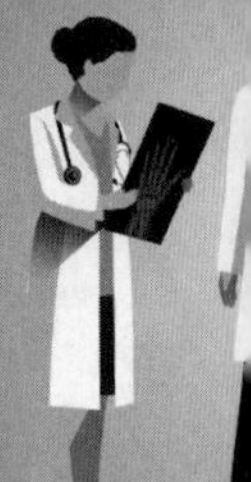

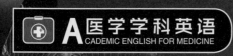

- To find more information about quoting and paraphrasing, you may refer to the following sources.
  1. Harris, R. A. 2001. Differences in quoting, paraphrasing and summarizing. Retrieved September 27, 2020, from Aquinas website.
  2. Kearney, V. 2022. Examples of summary, quotation and paraphrase. Retrieved August 14, 2022, from Owlcation website.

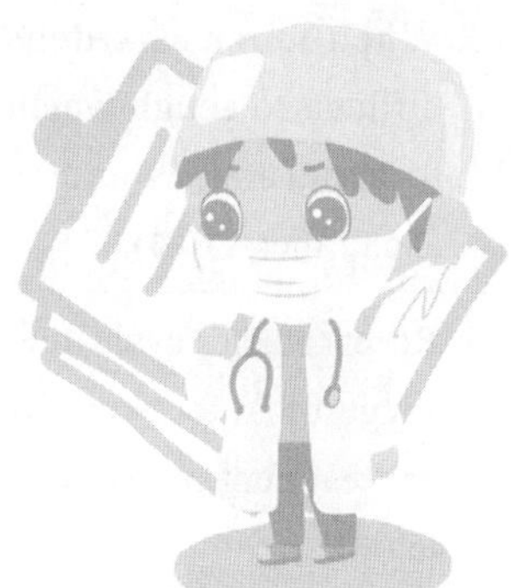

Unit 8

Medical Ethics

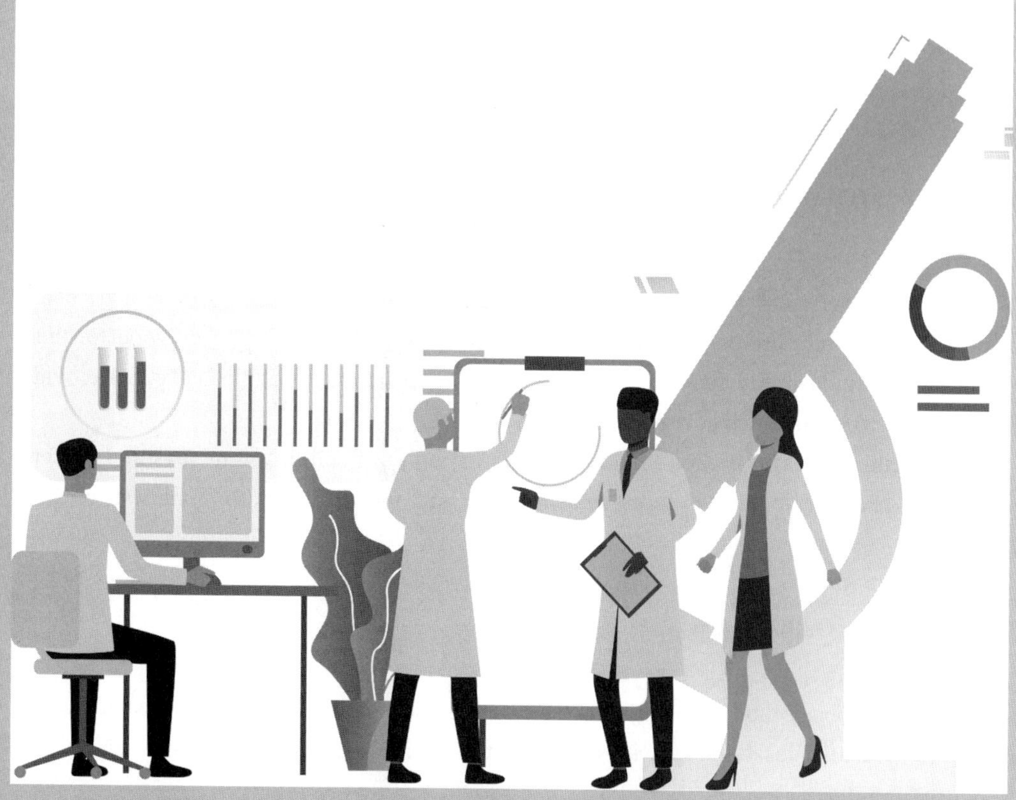

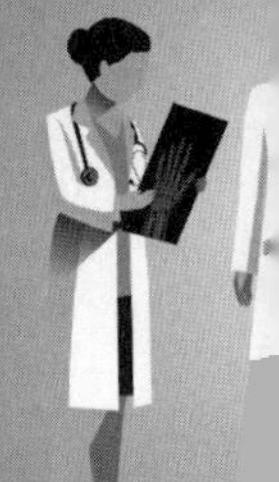

Part A Information Searching and Delivering

I. Surf on the Internet and find information about the following topics of medical ethics before class.

1. palliative care
2. organ donations
3. euthanasia
4. cloning
5. patient privacy

II. Make a presentation based on the information you've searched.

Part B Text Understanding

Passage 1 Introduction to Medical Ethics (Excerpt)

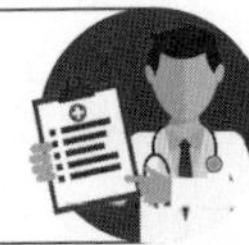

Ethics is the theory of moral behaviour and deals with the concepts of "good" and "bad". Medicine is an ethically driven profession due to the trust placed in doctors to do good for their patients and the responsibility that this brings. It is therefore paramount that medical ethics provide a high moral standard to which doctors must adhere.

Medical ethics are also needed to guide doctors through difficult decisions regarding patient care and to ensure they are always acting in accordance with the wishes and best interests of their patients.

The Hippocratic Oath

The moral responsibilities of being a doctor have long been recognised. The Hippocratic Oath, which dates back to at least 400 BC, is considered the earliest expression of medical ethics and reflects some of the pillars of medical ethics used today. The four basic pillars of medical ethics are beneficence, non-maleficence, justice, and autonomy. At a glance, these principles appear simple, and there are many examples of clearly unethical medical decisions. Yet ethical dilemmas are common within medicine, and there is not always an agreed-upon "right" decision.

Pillars of medical ethics 

1. The pillar of beneficence

The pillar of beneficence is about promoting the good of others. In medicine it means acting in a way that helps your patients. The most obvious example of this is providing up to date, evidence-based treatments to your patients with the aim of reducing their symptoms or treating their illness.

An extreme example of the principle of beneficence being neglected is the Tuskegee Syphilis Trial. It was carried out by the US Public Health Service from 1932 to observe the natural history of syphilis. In this trial, hundreds of African Americans who were found to have syphilis were told that they had "bad blood". They were offered free meals, health care and burial insurance if they took part in the trial. They were not fully informed that they had syphilis and were not offered any treatment even when penicillin was found to be effective in 1947.

The trial was only stopped in 1972 when an advisory panel found it unethical. These patients were known to have a disease that if untreated, can cause serious damage to the heart, nervous system and brain and can even cause death and were not given a known effective treatment. The doctors involved failed to help their patients, instead focusing on their research goals, which was a gross betrayal of research ethics and beneficence.

2. The pillar of non-maleficence

Non-maleficence refers to not causing harm to your patients. This principle spans a range of applications such as doctors maintaining medical competence and not giving patients treatments where the risks outweigh the benefits. It seems obvious that doctors would not want to harm their patients, yet there are countless examples of when this principle has been disregarded.

Harold Shipman was an infamous GP in England who qualified in 1970 and was found guilty and sent to prison for killing 15 of his patients and is suspected of killing hundreds more. He targeted elderly and vulnerable patients and gave them high-dose opiates ending their lives.

The Gosport War Memorial Hospital faced a similar scandal that involved the shortening of hundreds of lives starting in the late 1990s. Patients were again given high-dose painkillers without clinical indication.

These examples are incredibly shocking to all in the medical profession but demonstrate the

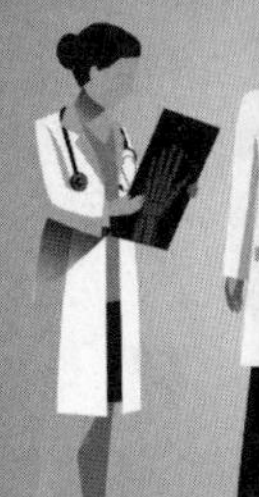

need for systems to protect patients from doctors who fail to uphold the ethical standards that they should. Non-maleficence and beneficence are usually balanced in that the risks or side effects of treatment should not outweigh the benefits. It is surprising how conflicting helping and not harming your patient can be.

3. The pillar of justice

The principle of justice refers to fairness within medicine and equal distribution of resources. It can be considered in terms of equality and equity of healthcare across patients.

Health equality refers to equal opportunity to access healthcare and means patients should not be discriminated against. Patients should be treated fairly regardless of groups such as gender, socioeconomic class, ethnicity, age etc. Patients who are all provided with the same services may still experience different outcomes due to barriers to certain patient groups accessing those services.

Equity refers to the fairness of outcome and means that those who are at a disadvantage to start with should be given greater support to compensate. Examples of health equity would include providing transport to a hospital for patients from low socioeconomic groups or improving staff training for treating people with disabilities. It could also involve identifying, for example, higher rates of smoking in certain geographical areas and thus providing more smoking cessation services in these areas.

Inequity within healthcare services tends to mean that those most likely to need healthcare are those that will struggle the most to access it. Health inequalities are unfair differences in health across groups in the population. There are many examples of health inequalities, but one example is the "social gradient" of health in England, where life expectancy increases as the level of social deprivation decreases.

4. The pillar of autonomy (self-determination)

The final pillar is autonomy and refers to a patient's right to make their own healthcare decisions. This is also known as self-determination. It means that patients can decide their own healthcare priorities, and it includes their right to refuse treatment. Doctors should inform and advise patients according to medical evidence; however, the final decision should always lie with the patient even if it goes against medical advice.

A common example is a Jehovah's Witness who may refuse a blood transfusion on religious grounds. This may seem medically unwise, but the patient has a right to refuse this treatment. Autonomy brings together many ethical challenges, including the areas of consent and capacity.

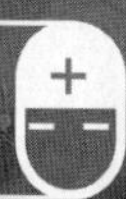

Final thoughts

The four pillars of medical ethics appear to be good moral standards for doctors to stand by. However, medical ethics are not always clear cut. Debate and disagreement around the end of life care, abortion and treating people without the capacity, for example, are likely to always exist. Knowing which option is the best for your patient is not always obvious.

As well as this, there are countless examples where medical ethics have unquestionably been broken and doctors have betrayed the trust placed in them by their patients. For these reasons, medical ethics must continue to be explored and debated. Moreover, doctors must continue to be held to the highest of standards to ensure that they are deserving of the trust placed in them.

Source: Melvin, H. 2020, October 30. Medical ethics: Ethical dilemmas in healthcare. *Medical Projects.*

I. Match the words with their definitions according to Passage 1.

____ 1. paramount	ⓐ a basic part or feature of a system, organization, belief, etc.
____ 2. pillar	ⓑ extremely startling, distressing, or offensive
____ 3. autonomy	ⓒ to include a large area or a lot of things
____ 4. outweigh	ⓓ well-known as being wicked or immoral
____ 5. shocking	ⓔ (of a crime, etc.) very obvious and unacceptable
____ 6. painkiller	ⓕ the result or effect of an action or event
____ 7. span	ⓖ having the greatest importance or significance
____ 8. infamous	ⓗ the ability to act and make decisions without being controlled by anyone else
____ 9. gross	ⓘ to be greater or more important than sth.
____ 10. outcome	ⓙ a medicine which reduces or removes pain

II. Read Passage 1 and answer the following questions.

1. What is the Hippocratic Oath?

____

2. What can you learn from the example of the Tuskegee Syphilis Trial?

____

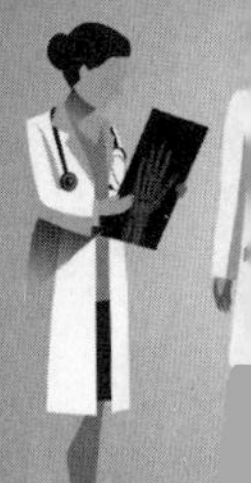

3. What do the examples of Harold Shipman and the Gosport War Memorial Hospital reveal?

____

4. What are equality and equity of healthcare across patients?

____

5. What is the author's attitude toward medical ethics?

____

Passage 2 Palliative Care—A Shifting Paradigm

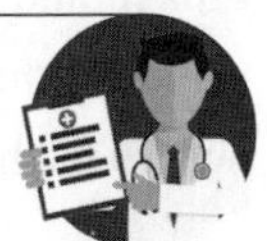

Palliative care focuses on relieving suffering and achieving the best possible quality of life for patients and their family caregivers. It involves the assessment and treatment of symptoms; support for decision making and assistance in matching treatments to informed patient and family goals; practical aid for patients and their family caregivers; mobilization of community resources to ensure a secure and safe living environment; and collaborative and seamless models of care across a range of care settings (i.e., hospital, home, nursing home, and hospice). Palliative care is provided both within the medicare hospice benefit (hospice palliative care) and outside it (nonhospice palliative care). Nonhospice palliative care is offered simultaneously with life-prolonging and curative therapies for persons living with serious, complex, and life-threatening illness. Hospice palliative care becomes appropriate when curative treatments are no longer beneficial, when the burdens of these treatments exceed their benefits, or when patients are entering the last weeks to months of life.

Comprehensive palliative care services integrate the expertise of a team of providers from different disciplines to address the complex needs of seriously ill patients and their families. Members of a palliative care team typically include professionals from medicine, nursing, and social work, with additional support from chaplaincy and professionals in nutrition, rehabilitation, pharmacy, and other professional disciplines, as needed. These programs are now available at more than 80% of large US hospitals (those with more than 300 beds), where most Americans receive their care during complex and advanced illness.

Despite the increasing availability of palliative care services in US hospitals and the body of evidence showing the great distress to patients caused by symptoms of the illness, the burdens on family caregivers, and the overuse of costly, ineffective therapies during advanced chronic illness, the use of palliative care services by physicians for their patients remains low. Physicians tend to perceive palliative care as the alternative to life-prolonging or curative care—what we do when there is nothing more that we can do—rather than as a simultaneously delivered adjunct to disease-

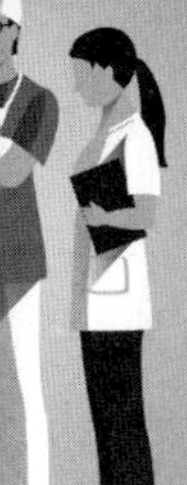

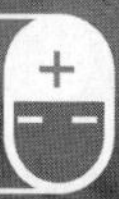

focused treatment.

In this issue of the *Journal,* Temel and colleagues challenge this prevailing notion of palliative care by presenting the results of a randomized, controlled trial of early palliative care in addition to standard oncologic care for patients with newly diagnosed metastatic non-small-cell lung cancer. A total of 151 subjects were recruited and enrolled in the study at a single academic thoracic oncology practice. Health-related quality of life and mood were measured at baseline and at 12 weeks. In addition to standard oncologic care, patients in the intervention group met with a palliative care clinician at the time of enrollment and at least monthly thereafter. As compared with the standard care group, the intervention group had better quality of life, lower rates of depression, and a 2.7-month survival benefit.

The results of this study show that palliative care is appropriate and potentially beneficial when it is introduced at the time of diagnosis of a serious or life-limiting illness—at the same time as all other appropriate and beneficial medical therapies are initiated. The fact that palliative care improved quality-of-life outcomes is consistent with the results of other studies of both nonhospice and hospice palliative care. The substantial survival advantage observed, though it is supported by other recent studies, requires replication.

The specific components of the study's palliative care intervention remain unspecified and hence may not be easily reproducible in other practice settings. For example, the salutary effect of additional time with and attention from health care providers and physicians, as opposed to a specific benefit derived from palliative care itself, was not assessed and is a limitation of the study. The reasons for the 2.7-month survival benefit in the palliative care group—a benefit that is equivalent to that achieved with a response to standard chemotherapy regimens—are unknown but may result from effective treatment of depression, improved management of symptoms, or a reduction in the need for hospitalization. The current study was not designed to address these important questions. Despite these limitations, Temel and colleagues are to be commended for overcoming many of the challenges and barriers to conducting a randomized trial of a palliative care intervention.

Future studies of palliative care must begin to test and identify the actual components of palliative care that are provided and received. Such methodologic rigor is necessary to establish the evidence for best practice. Studies of other disease populations beyond patients with cancer and in other settings (e.g., long-term care) are also necessary to identify the ways in which palliative care can be appropriately delivered in diverse patient populations and settings. Finally, although studies have shown that palliative care programs reduce hospital expenditures, additional studies examining the effect of palliative care on overall health care costs need to be undertaken.

The study by Temel et al. represents an important step in confirming the beneficial outcomes of a simultaneous care model that provides both palliative care and disease-specific therapies beginning at the time of diagnosis. This study is an example of research that shifts a long-held

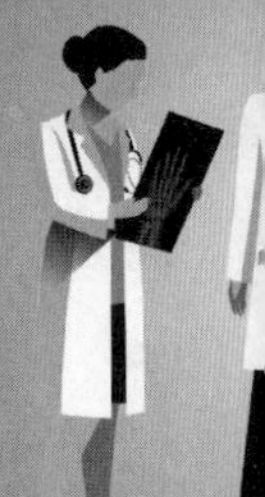

paradigm that has limited access to palliative care to patients who were predictably and clearly dying. The new approach recognizes that life-threatening illness, whether it can be cured or controlled, carries with it significant burdens of suffering for patients and their families and that this suffering can be effectively addressed by modern palliative care teams. Perhaps unsurprisingly, reducing patients' misery may help them live longer. We now have both the means and the knowledge to make palliative care an essential and routine component of evidence-based, high-quality care for the management of serious illness.

Source: Amy, S. et al. 2010. Palliative care—a shifting paradigm. *The New England Journal of Medicine, 363*: 781-782.

I. Match the words with their definitions according to Passage 2.

____ 1. palliative	ⓐ amount of money spent
____ 2. paradigm	ⓑ branch of knowledge
____ 3. seamless	ⓒ (formal or technical) a typical example or pattern of sth.
____ 4. discipline	ⓓ a regulated system, as of medication, diet, or exercise, used to promote health or treat illness or injury
____ 5. issue	ⓔ smoothly continuous or uniform in quality
____ 6. salutary	ⓕ the fact of being careful and paying great attention to detail
____ 7. regimen	ⓖ (medical) a medicine or medical treatment that reduces pain without curing its cause
____ 8. commend	ⓗ (of an experience) having a good effect on sb./sth., though often seeming unpleasant
____ 9. rigor	ⓘ one of a regular series of magazines or newspapers
____ 10. expenditure	ⓙ to praise sb./sth., especially publicly

II. Read Passage 2 and answer the following questions.

1. According to the passage, what does "a shifting paradigm" in the title mean?

____

2. What is palliative care?

____

3. What is the current status of palliative care?

____

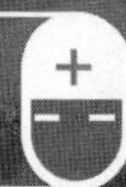

4. When should palliative care be conducted according to the passage?

____

5. What does the role of palliative care play in treating a patient with cancer in your opinion?

____

Passage 3 A Genetically Augmented Future

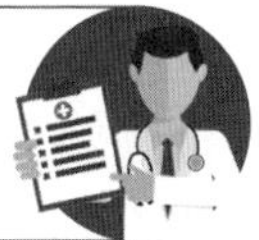

The year is 2030. Gene therapy to insert the DNA sequence for dystrophin has been approved by regulators and is commonly used in children with Duchenne Muscular Dystrophy (DMD), a disorder linked to the X chromosome. Evidence shows that the intervention increases muscle mass in anyone who receives it. The treatment is widely available, but very expensive.

Alex, a slender adolescent, walks into a physician's office, accompanied by well-to-do parents. Alex does not have DMD, but wants to be stronger. Exercise is not providing enough benefits, and anabolic steroids have too many side effects. Alex is adamant about wanting dystrophin gene therapy and accurately cites its risks and benefits. Alex's parents are willing to pay for the treatment.

The cure for DMD described previously represents a cherished goal for gene therapy, and there is a lot of public support for fixing such heritable disorders in this way. Yet Alex's request raises a host of questions.

We do not know why Alex wants to be stronger. Alex could have a milder form of muscular dystrophy or, if female, could be a carrier who experiences milder symptoms of DMD. Alex might have some other cause of muscle weakness—or might want to be stronger for the sake of appearance, or to be more competitive in athletics. As is the case for many medical interventions, the potential uses of this therapy go beyond the specific disease for which it was developed. Possible applications range from treating milder disease to improving human characteristics—a continuum that could lack clear boundaries.

Let's assume that Alex does not have a diagnosed physical problem and wants the therapy simply to become stronger. The main debate about using medical interventions for such bodily enhancements focuses on the extent to which they give individuals an advantage over other people. A 2017 report by the US National Academies on gene editing in humans captures the debate well.

The authors summarize surveys that show most people disapprove of using gene therapy to improve a person's physical and intellectual characteristics. The public tends to honour narratives of success based on personal diligence, or even accident of birth, over traits that can

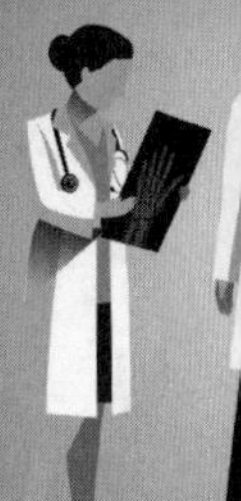

be purchased. This preference touches on a larger issue: the extent to which uses of gene therapy would exacerbate social inequality. If there is a widespread perception that this would be the result, society might try to limit its use to the few people who genuinely need it to treat their disease. Or there might be an effort to make such therapies available to all who want them.

Back to Alex in the world of 2030. Assuming that the US Food and Drug Administration's regulations are still the same, physicians would be free to use the approved DMD intervention for any purpose. After all, many medicines are legally prescribed for reasons that have nothing to do with their original indication. So what should happen? How hard should a physician try to understand the source of Alex's desire to be stronger?

Alex's wish might be a product of the social and cultural environment. The request might reflect issues with self-image. The desire to be stronger could reveal a psychological problem that needs to be resolved. Or a physician could conclude that Alex is suffering, thereby making the case for gene therapy more compelling. For example, medical and surgical interventions are sometimes prescribed to prevent or relieve psychological distress in children or young people who are abnormally short or who have potentially stigmatizing physical features. It is important to ensure that Alex understands and agrees to the therapy, but in the end, it can be hard to ascertain the source of a person's desire for a given treatment—especially if the person is an adolescent.

Are Alex's parents wrong to support their child's desire? Perhaps they are putting undue pressure on Alex. Perhaps they want to alleviate Alex's distress. Perhaps they are just indulgent. Society's default position is that parents should have the last say in such matters because they are assumed to care more for their children than does anyone else. Parents have a responsibility for shaping their children's future, creating opportunities and drilling into them all sorts of values. Parents are largely free to pursue their vision for their children's lives, unless those actions are illegal or constitute abuse or neglect.

So what is the physician to do? Assuming that gene therapy for enhancement has not been outlawed, he or she can and should turn to medical ethics and the goals of medicine for guidance. Respect for persons—a fundamental principle of medical ethics—would direct the physician to attempt to discover more about what is driving the patient and their parents' wishes, and to ensure that they understand what is at stake and that their expectations are realistic. If the decision to proceed was made to relieve suffering, and with the adolescent's informed assent and the parents' permission, pursuing the goals of medicine would lead the physician to use the therapy to confer only traits within the normal range of human characteristics.

Ultimately, the ethics of enhancement are intertwined with views of fairness. Concerns about equity should lead society to develop guidelines for gene therapy to avoid a nightmare future in which a group of privileged people becomes stronger, smarter and more beautiful than the rest. But because drawing lines between treatment and enhancement is difficult, the more likely and more unsettling scenario is that physicians will be left to rely on their own ethical commitments to decide when to use gene therapy.

Source: Clayton, E. w. 2019, January 14. A genetically augmented future. *Scientific American.*

I. Match the words with their definitions according to Passage 3.

____ 1. adamant	a impossible to persuade, or unwilling to change an opinion or decision
____ 2. cite	b an artificial form of a natural chemical substance which is used for treating particular medical conditions
____ 3. honour	c to make sth. no longer legal
____ 4. steroid	d to make sth. worse, especially a disease or problem
____ 5. trait	e willing to allow someone, especially a child, to do or have whatever they want, even if this is not good for them
____ 6. exacerbate	f a description of how things might happen in the future
____ 7. undue	g more than right or proper
____ 8. indulgent	h to give the exact words of something that has been written, especially in order to support an opinion or prove an idea
____ 9. outlaw	i a particular characteristic, quality, or tendency that sb. or sth. has
____ 10. scenario	j to give public praise, an award or a title to sb. for sth. they have done

II. Read Passage 3 and answer the following questions.

1. Why does Alex's request raise a host of questions?
   ____
2. Why do most people show disapproval to gene editing?
   ____
3. What will the physician do with gene therapy in the future?
   ____
4. What could be the undesirable results of gene therapy?
   ____
5. What is your opinion toward gene therapy?
   ____

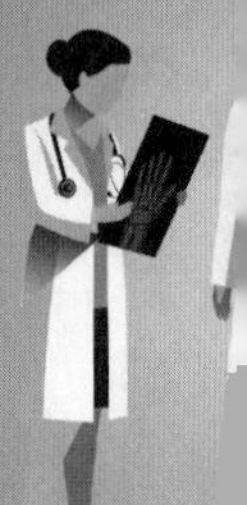

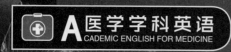

III. Read the three passages comprehensively and answer the following questions.

1. What do the three passages discuss in common?

____

2. What are the focuses of three passages respectively?

____

3. In your opinion, what attributes should a good doctor have?

____

4. Write a short passage of about 100 words to synthesize the information of the three passages.

____

____

____

____

____

Part C | Integrated Exercises

I. Read the words below, and pay attention to the pronunciation. Use the scale below (1, 2, 3) to give yourself a score for each word. Try to consult your dictionary for the words with score 1.

❶ I don't understand this word.

❷ I understand this word when I see it or hear it, but I don't know how to use it.

❸ I know this word and can use it in my own speaking and writing.

Academic words

□ adamant	□ autonomy	□ beneficence	□ beneficial
□ betray	□ capture	□ cite	□ collaborative
□ commend	□ compensate	□ comprehensive	□ confer
□ conflicting	□ deprivation	□ dilemma	□ discipline
□ discriminate	□ disregard	□ equity	□ ethically
□ exacerbate	□ expenditure	□ gross	□ ground

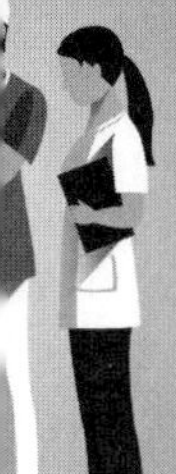

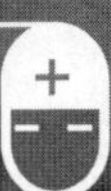

☐ incredibly	☐ indulgent	☐ inequality	☐ infamous
☐ insert	☐ issue	☐ justice	☐ maleficence
☐ misery	☐ mobilization	☐ outcome	☐ outlaw
☐ outweigh	☐ paradigm	☐ paramount	☐ pillar
☐ predictably	☐ randomized	☐ recruit	☐ relieve
☐ replication	☐ reproducible	☐ rigor	☐ salutary
☐ scandal	☐ scenario	☐ seamless	☐ secure
☐ shift	☐ simultaneously	☐ span	☐ undue
☐ unquestionably	☐ unspecified	☐ uphold	☐ vulnerable

Discipline-specific words

☐ abortion	☐ anabolic	☐ chromosome	☐ curative
☐ dose	☐ dystrophin	☐ dystrophy	☐ genetically
☐ heritable	☐ hospice	☐ indication	☐ intervention
☐ mass	☐ muscular	☐ oncological	☐ opiate
☐ painkiller	☐ palliative	☐ penicillin	☐ regimen
☐ rehabilitation	☐ survival	☐ syphilis	☐ thoracic
☐ transfusion			

II. Match each word in the box with the group of words that regularly occur in academic writing.

fix	raise	capture	alleviate	confer
uphold	betray	recruit	insert	resolve

1. ______________ one's attention / one's interest / one's heart
2. ______________ money / one's awareness / one's voice
3. ______________ pain / poverty / symptom
4. ______________ soldiers / members / volunteers
5. ______________ a dispute / a conflict / a crisis
6. ______________ a comment / a thermometer / a key
7. ______________ a title / a degree / an honour
8. ______________ one's friends / one's country / one's emotions
9. ______________ a decision / a law / a principle
10. ______________ a machine / a mistake / the fault

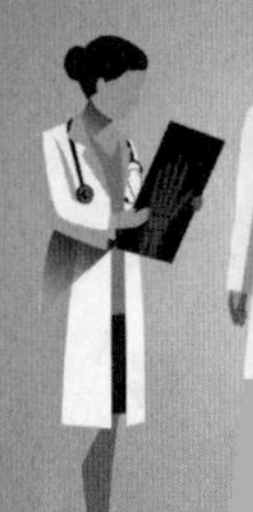

III. Study the members of the word families in the table below. Try to work out the meaning in each case according to its prefix or suffix.

The members of a word family	Chinese definitions
ethic, ethical, ethically, unethical	伦理标准、伦理的、伦理上地、不道德的
just, justify, justice	
indicate, indication, indicator	
credit, credible, incredible, incredibly	
deprive, deprived, deprivation	
abort, abortion, abortionist	
equal, equality, inequality	
question, questionable, questionably, unquestionably	
vulnerable, vulnerably, vulnerability	
anabolite, anabolic, anabolism	
discriminate, discrimination, discriminatory	
benefit, beneficial, beneficiary	
random, randomly, randomness, randomize	
predict, prediction, predictable, predictably	
misery, miserable, miserably	
thorax, thoracic, thoracotomy	
mobile, mobility, mobilize, mobilization	
reproduce, reproductive, reproducible	
specify, specified, unspecified	
dystrophy, dystrophic, dystrophin	

IV. Complete each sentence below with a word from the table above.

1. This situation imposed on humankind a responsibility to develop ________ sound systems of medical governance. (ethic)
2. A bruit is usually detected with a stethoscope and is an ________ of arterial blockage. (indicate)
3. Eating healthily has always been an ________ important aspect of keeping the body, and mind clean and healthy. (credit)
4. Underage ________ can be very harmful to a girl, both physically and mentally. (abort)
5. The billions of bacteria and other microscopic critters that live in the mouth ________ influence the health of teeth and gums. (question)
6. The failure to promote and protect human rights increases ________ and can drive HIV epidemics. (vulnerable)
7. It is really exciting that this new class of treatment seems to have ________ effects on the cardiovascular system. (benefit)
8. Conventional drugs are usually tested in healthy volunteers, as toxicity is usually limited and ________. (predict)
9. The measures taken include clinical management, vector control, and social ________. (mobile)
10. Aging is an extremely complex, multi-factorial process influenced by the environment, disease, genetic and other ________ effects. (specify)

V. Choose the word in each list that is not a synonym for the underlined word.

1. <u>dilemma</u>
   A. predicament　B. quandary　C. solution　D. plight
2. <u>enhancement</u>
   A. improvement　B. boost　C. betterment　D. decline
3. <u>secure</u>
   A. endangered　B. safe　C. shielded　D. protected
4. <u>collaborative</u>
   A. cooperative　B. separate　C. combined　D. jointly
5. <u>simultaneously</u>
   A. concurrently　B. synchronously　C. diachronically　D. meanwhile
6. <u>comprehensive</u>
   A. specific　B. inclusive　C. thorough　D. overall
7. <u>replication</u>
   A. reproduction　B. copy　C. duplication　D. archetype

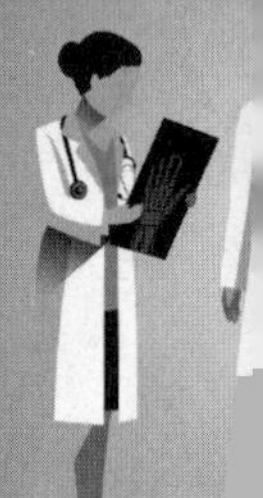

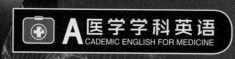

8. shift
   A. change　　B. remain　　C. switch　　D. alter
9. confirm
   A. prove　　B. contradict　　C. validate　　D. verify
10. heritable
   A. familial　　B. hereditary　　C. genetic　　D. acquired

VI. Read the following expressions and sentence patterns aloud and analyze the formality of the structures used.

Target sentence patterns

1. It is therefore paramount that medical ethics provide a high moral standard **to** which doctors must **adhere**.
2. Medical ethics are also needed to guide doctors through difficult decisions regarding patient care and to ensure they are always acting **in accordance with** the wishes and best interests of their patients.
3. **At a glance**, these principles appear simple, and there are many examples of clearly unethical medical decisions.
4. This principle spans **a range of** applications such as doctors maintaining medical competence and not giving patients treatments where the risks outweigh the benefits.
5. Harold Shipman was an infamous GP in England who qualified in 1970 and was found guilty and **sent to prison** for killing 15 of his patients and **is suspected of** killing hundreds more.
6. It can be considered **in terms of** equality and equity of healthcare across patients.
7. Equity refers to the fairness of outcome and means that those who are **at a disadvantage** to start with should be given greater support to compensate.
8. However, the final decision should always **lie with** the patient even if it **goes against** medical advice.
9. The four pillars of medical ethics **appear to** be good moral standards for doctors to **stand by**.
10. Moreover, doctors must continue to be held to the highest of standards to ensure that they **are deserving of** the trust placed in them.
11. Physicians tend to **perceive** palliative care **as** the alternative to life-prolonging or curative care—what we do when there is nothing more that we can do—rather than as a simultaneously delivered **adjunct to** disease-focused treatment.

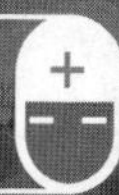

12. For example, the salutary effect of additional time with and attention from health care providers and physicians, **as opposed to** a specific benefit derived from palliative care itself, was not assessed and is a limitation of the study.
13. The reasons for the 2.7-month survival benefit in the palliative care group—a benefit that **is equivalent to** that achieved with a **response to** standard chemotherapy regimens—are unknown but may **result from** effective treatment of depression, improved management of symptoms, or a reduction in the need for hospitalization.
14. Yet Alex's request raises **a host of** questions.
15. Alex might have some other cause of muscle weakness—or might want to be stronger **for the sake of** appearance, or to be more competitive in athletics.
16. **As is the case for** many medical interventions, the potential uses of this therapy **go beyond** the specific disease for which it was developed.
17. The main debate about using medical interventions for such bodily enhancements **focuses on** the extent to which they **give individuals an advantage over** other people.
18. This preference **touches on** a larger issue: the extent to which uses of gene therapy would exacerbate social inequality.
19. If **there is a widespread perception that** this would be the result, society might try to limit its use to the few people who genuinely need it to treat their disease.
20. Perhaps they are **putting** undue **pressure on** Alex.
21. Society's default position is that parents should **have the last say** in such matters because they are assumed to care more for their children than does anyone else.
22. Parents **have a responsibility for** shaping their children's future, creating opportunities and **drilling into** them all sorts of values.
23. He or she can and should **turn to** medical ethics and the goals of medicine **for** guidance.
24. Respect for persons—a fundamental principle of medical ethics—would direct the physician to attempt to discover more about what is driving the patient and their parents' wishes, and to ensure that they understand what **is at stake** and that their expectations are realistic.
25. Ultimately, the ethics of enhancement **are intertwined with** views of fairness.

VII. For each of the sentences below, write a new sentence as similar as possible in meaning to the original one, but as formal as possible in style.

1. The mouse turned out to be vulnerable to a lot of infections, but its susceptibility to herpes simplex had not been tested.

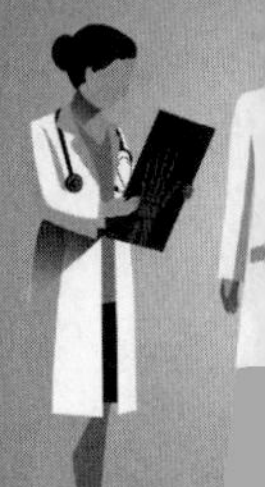

2. Household pesticides must be handled according to the label instructions.

3. The diagnosis is important in organizing and planning treatment.

4. For these types of injuries, topical oxygen may be helpful as an additional means to surgery or other forms of standard wound care.

5. Our minds have a number of ways to shield us from information that we have learned to view as painful.

6. People usually think keeping optimistic can promote health.

7. If we compare the health risks, obesity is equal to smoking a pack of cigarettes a day!

8. Old age brings with it a number of physical woes, and among the most common is hearing loss.

9. Who will make the final decision when doctors and parents disagree about a child's medical treatment?

10. Medicine is closely connected with warfare.

VIII. Translate the following sentences by using the following words and phrases. Make sure that your English sentences are different from the Chinese versions in terms of structures or orders, but as formal as possible. Then compare yours with your partner's according to the criteria: Whose version is more different and more formal?

1. 任何医生如果在处理患者时不遵守指南规定，其收入将会按比例减少。(adhere to)

____

2. 她对该医学领域一无所知，这显然对她极其不利。(at a disadvantage)

____

3. 医生一眼就看出那个孩子染上了麻疹。(at a glance)

____

4. 美国疾病控制中心指出，过去的十年里总共在 11 个国家出现过 196 个人类受感病例。(a total of)

____

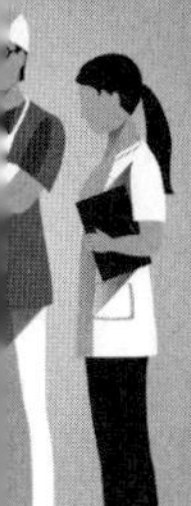

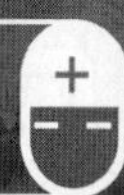

5. 与生理成瘾相反，患成瘾性疾病的重大潜在风险并不适用于每一个人。(as opposed to)

____

6. 医生认为她不宜从事正常工作。(carry out)

____

7. 目前应对霍乱暴发往往是反应性的。(response to)

____

8. 公众健康正处在生死攸关的境地，是时候给予美国食品药物管理局充足经费了。(be at stake)

____

9. 这种流行病将给全球谷物和其他粮食价格带来压力。(put pressure on)

____

10. 以影像为引导的医学为医师提供了抗癌的优势。(give... an advantage over...)

____

Part D | Academic Skills

Academic Listening Skill

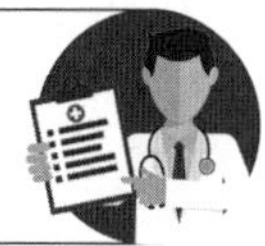

Summarizing

Summarizing is one of the vital skills when we listen. A summary should cover the main idea, major events, and important details. To work out the summary of the text, listeners should pay attention to the first sentence and the ending sentence. Besides, listeners should notice the signal words. At last, the change of the subtopic counts when you summarize. In other words, while listening, listeners should pay attention to when the speaker shifts from one subtopic to another. And then they should go on to seize related details under each subtopic.

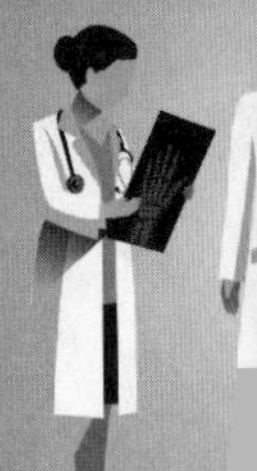

Listening 1

Word bank

1. ultimately	finally, after everything else has been done or considered
2. valid	officially acceptable
3. cast	a hard protective case that is put over your arm, leg etc. because the bone is broken
4. alternative	different from the one you have and can be used instead
5. carpal	relating to the wrist bones
6. tunnel	a long passage of a people's body
7. factually	based on facts or relating to facts

I. The passage you are going to listen to contains three points when a doctor wants to obtain a valid consent. Listen and write down the first sentence of each point.

1. ______________________________
2. ______________________________
3. ______________________________

II. Listen to the passage and decide whether the following statements are true (T) or false (F).

1. A patient can voluntarily choose to proceed with a treatment or not. ( )
2. A physician doesn't need to obtain valid consent before fulfilling a treatment. ( )
3. A physician is responsible for helping the patient choose a treatment plan. ( )
4. Patients' capacities of understanding the nature of the proposed treatment vary. ( )
5. A physician needs to provide patients with information about the expected benefits of a treatment. ( )

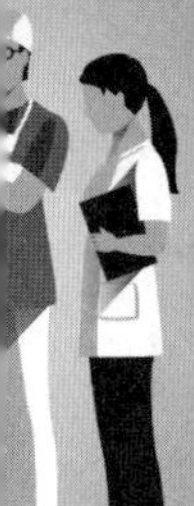

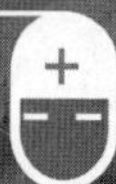

Listening 2

Word bank

1. first-ever	never having happened or been experienced before
2. identical	similar in every detail
3. deceased	no longer living
4. compatible	able to exist or be used together without causing problems
5. negative	no evidence of the medical condition or substance that you are looking for
6. recipient	a person who receives sth.
7. downside	the disadvantages or less positive aspects of sth.
8. pathogen	a thing that causes disease
9. immunosuppressive	of or relating to a substance that lowers the body's normal immune response and induces immunosuppression
10. oppress	to subdue or suppress
11. susceptible	very likely to be influenced, harmed or affected by sb./sth.
12. exploit	to treat a person or situation as an opportunity to gain an advantage for yourself
13. violate	to disturb or not respect sb.'s peace, privacy, etc.

I. Listen to the passage and choose the best answer to each of the questions.

1 What is the proper title for this passage?

A Why do we transplant organs?

B How do we transplant organs?

C Organ transplants and ethics.

D Advantages and disadvantages of organ transplantation.

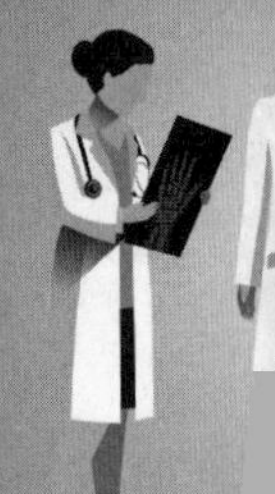

❷ What will facilitate the process of organ transplant according to the passage?

Ⓐ 3-D printing of organs.

Ⓑ Stem cell research.

Ⓒ Organ farms in labs.

Ⓓ All the above.

II. Listen to the passage and answer the following questions.

1. What is organ transplant according to the passage?

   1) An organ transplant is the ____.

   2) Transplant can ____.

   3) The donated organ can be from ________________ or ________________________.

2. What are the factors taken into consideration when matching donor organs to receivers?

   1) ____

   2) ____

   3) ____

   4) ____

   5) ____

3. The downsides of organ transplant.

   1) Sometimes the recipient's immune system will ________________________.

   2) Receivers are given immunosuppressive drugs.

      a. Too __________ drugs: the patient ________________________________.

      b. Too __________ drugs: the patient ________________________________.

4. What are the ethical issues surrounding organ transplants according to the passage?

   1) Living donors potentially ______________.

   2) ____ even though the operation might not be a success.

   3) "________________________"

   If the rich can buy organs of living donors, this has great ________________________ and ________________.

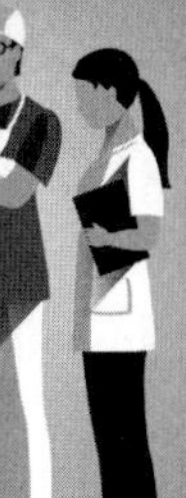

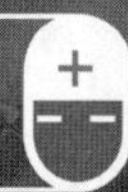

Academic Reading Skill

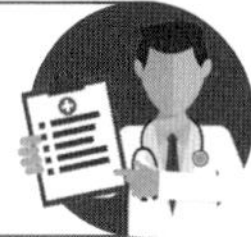

Tables and Figures

Both tables and figures belong to visual elements, which are useful for presenting data and augmenting ideas. They help readers understand a complicated process or visualize trends in the data. Tables and figures are different in their form and function. Tables are graphics that use row-and-column structures to organize information, whereas figures include illustrations or images other than tables. Elements of table include numbers, titles, headings, body, borders and notes. Figures include numbers, titles, image, legends and notes. Readers should note that every table and figure has a caption, too. As for caption, it is a short block of the text that gives information of the table or figure, which includes number, title, and other appropriate explanatory information, as shown below.

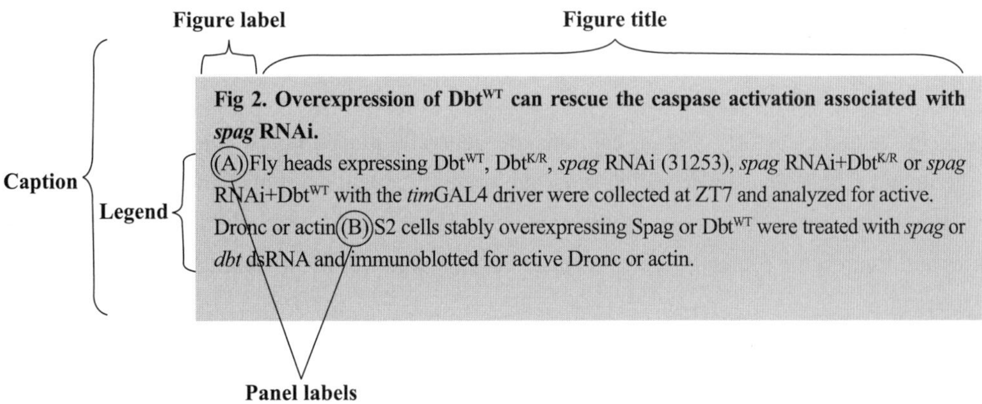

Fig 2. Overexpression of Dbt^{WT} can rescue the caspase activation associated with *spag* RNAi.
(A) Fly heads expressing Dbt^{WT}, $Dbt^{K/R}$, *spag* RNAi (31253), *spag* RNAi+$Dbt^{K/R}$ or *spag* RNAi+Dbt^{WT} with the *tim*GAL4 driver were collected at ZT7 and analyzed for active. Dronc or actin (B) S2 cells stably overexpressing Spag or Dbt^{WT} were treated with *spag* or *dbt* dsRNA and immunoblotted for active Dronc or actin.

Source: Means, J. C., Venkatesan, A., Gerdes, B., Fan, J.-Y., Bjes, E. S. & Price, J. L. 2015. Drosophila spaghetti and doubletime link the circadian clock and light to caspases, apoptosis and tauopathy. *PLoS Genet, 11*(5): e1005171.

Each table is numbered with Arabic numerals sequentially, like Table 1, Table 2, Table 3. And each table has a clear, descriptive and concise title. Table caption needs to be placed above the table since we read tables from the top down. Table has several types of headings: *stub headings, column headings, column spanners and table spanners.*

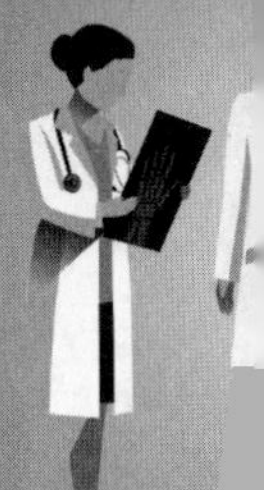

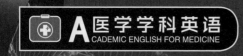

- Stub headings describe the lefthand column, which usually lists major independent variables.
- Column headings describe entries below them. Column headings only apply to just *one* column.
- Column spanners are different because they apply to *two or more* columns and each column has its exclusive column heading.
- Table spanners cover the entire width of the table.

To fulfill clarity, the abovementioned headings need separating by borders and lines. All the information reported in the intersections of rows and columns constitutes the main part of the table which is the body. In terms of note, there are three types: *general notes, specific notes and probability notes*.

- General notes explain, qualify or provide information about the table as a whole. Put explanations of abbreviations, symbols, etc.
- Specific notes explain, qualify or provide information about a particular column, row, or individual entry.
- Probability notes provide the reader with the results of the tests for statistical significance.

Each figure is numbered with Arabic numerals, too, like Figure 1, Figure 2, etc. It also has a descriptive and clear title. Figure captions are generally placed below the figures. Body refers to the image. The legends, also called keys, are used to explain symbols, styles, patterns, shading or colors in the image. Notes clarify the content of the figure. Readers should notice that both in tables and figures, the source of the data or the visual image will be provided if they are not created by the author.

For any figure, or table, the primary thing readers should do is to look at the headings and units used. This will tell readers a lot about what is being represented in the data. If a line in a figure says "years" then readers figure out it could be sort of timeline. If a heading says "percentage who earns over 40,000 RMB per year" then readers know that in this table column there will be a list of percentages, and they are about a group of people whose income is over 40,000RMB each year. When reading a table, readers can read from left to right and then from top to bottom, and read across all the spanners and column headings for one column before moving on to the next.

Besides, the caption number is also referred to and discussed within the body text, which are often described as "See Figure 9 for a detailed schematic", or "The test results are summarized in Table 1".

 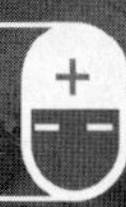

In conclusion, while doing academic reading of tables and figures, it is essential to take care of the details and remember tracing back to the body text to interpret relevant tables and figures.

I. Read each of the following tables and figure, and find out what element is missing.

1. What element is missing in the table below?

____

Table 8-1

Predominant term in ethics	Predominant term in research	Definition
Voluntary active euthanasia	Euthanasia	When a person (generally a physician) administers a medication, such as a sedative and neuromuscular relaxant, to intentionally end a patient's life with the mentally competent patient's **explicit request**
Involuntary active euthanasia	Ending a life without explicit patient request	When a physician or someone else administers a medication, such as sedative and neuromuscular relaxant, or other intervention, to intentionally end a patient's life but **without the mentally competent patient's request**
Nonvoluntary active euthanasia	Ending a life without explicit patient request	When a physician or someone else administers a medication, such as sedative and neuromuscular relaxant, or other intervention, to intentionally end a patient's life with a **noncompetent patient** who could not give informed consent because the patient is a child or has Alzheimer disease or other condition that compromises decision-making capacity
Physician-assisted suicide or physician-assisted death	Physician-assisted suicide	When the physician provides medication or a prescription to a patient at his or her **explicit request** with the understanding that the patient intends to use the medications to end his or her life

Source: Emanuel, E. et al. 2016. Attitudes and practices of euthanasia and physician-assisted suicide in the United States, Canada, and Europe. *JAMA, 316*(1): 79-90.

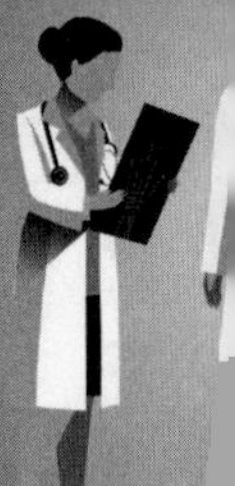

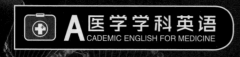

2. What element is missing in the table below?

____

Table 8-2 Number of CRISPR-Related Scientific Publications (2011–2018)

Year	Number
2011	87
2012	137
2013	300
2014	670
2015	1,457
2016	2,594
2017	3,738
2018	3,917
Total	**12,900**

Source: CRS analysis of data on scientific publications from Scopus as of November 20, 2018.

3. What element is missing in the figure below?

____

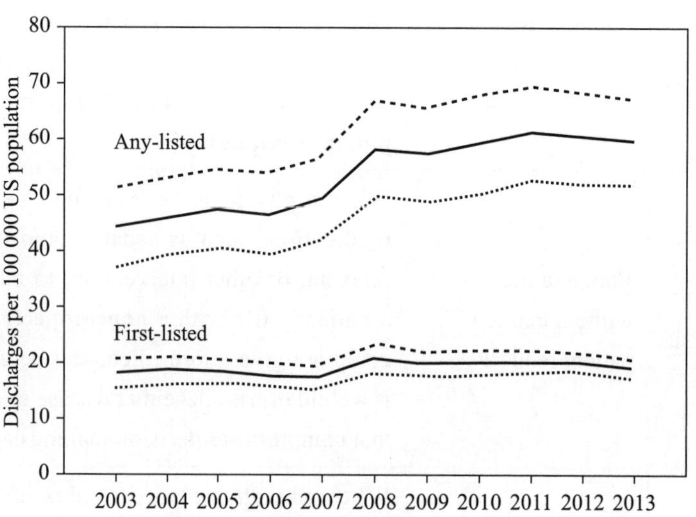

Figure 8-1

Source: Malarcher, C. A. et al. 2017. Hospitalizations for Crohn's Disease—United States (2003–2013). CDC. Retrieved January 15, 2023, from CDC website.

II. Read the following figure, and answer the questions below.

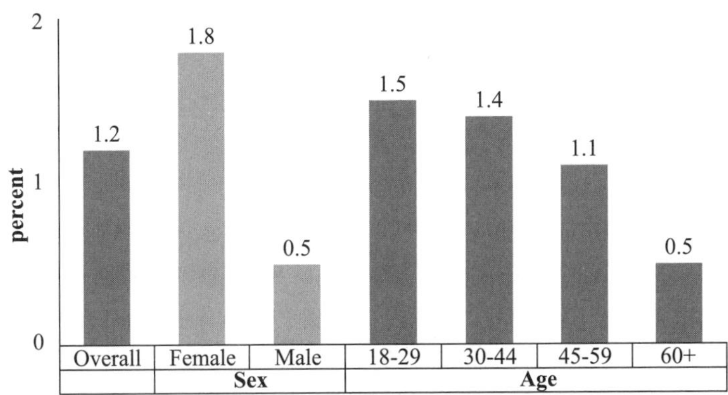

Figure 8-2 Past Year Prevalence of Obsessive-Compulsive Disorder Among US Adults (2001–2003) Data from National Comorbidity Survey Replication (NCS-R)

Source: National Institute of Mental Health, Obsessive-Compulsive Disorder (OCD)

1. What do the X-axis and Y-axis represent respectively?

____

____

____

2. What information is conveyed with regard to the light blue columns?

____

____

____

3. What information is conveyed with regard to the dark blue columns?

____

____

____

➢ To find more information about tables and figures, you may refer to the following sources.

1. Purdue Online Writing Lab. 2020. Tables and figures. Retrieved August 30, 2020, from Purdue Online Writing Lab website.
2. Cocas & Whittall. 2020. Figure caption guidelines. Retrieved August 30, 2020, from Santa Clara University website.
3. The College of Engineering, Utah State University. 2020. Additional resources: Tables and figures. Retrieved August 30, 2020, from the College of Engineering, Utah State University website.
4. Last, S. 2020. Figures and tables. Retrieved September 2, 2020, from Pressbooks website.

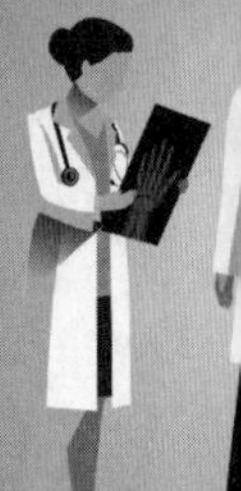

Academic Writing Skill

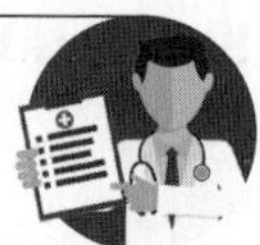

Summarizing

Compared with quoting and paraphrasing, summarizing is used when you don't have to provide the level of detail that the original writer did. **Summarizing** involves expressing the main idea of the source in your own general overview. So summaries mostly include the main point(s), and leave out details or examples that may distract the reader from the most important information, and they simplify complex arguments, grammar and vocabulary.

Although both paraphrasing and summarizing allow you to show your understanding and interpretation of a text with your own words, there are differences between paraphrasing and summarizing:

Paraphrasing	Summarizing
• clarify the source precisely • reword the source to match the original meaning • use details • approximately the same length, though often slightly shorter than the source	• condense the source briefly • sum up the source to give a general introduction • leave out details • significantly shorter than the source

When you summarize a text, you can follow the following steps:

1. Read the text and underline the key words, main ideas and supporting points;
2. Write down the words you underlined;
3. Write down main ideas in one or two sentences without looking at the source;
4. For each supporting point, write one to two sentence summaries in your own words;
5. Combine all written sentences into a paragraph;
6. Proofread your summary to check errors or repetitions;
7. Cite in order to avoid plagiarism.

To sum up, when incorporating sources into your writing, you should read them thoroughly to form a certain connection with your writing, so you can choose the sources that deserve being quoted directly, restate the sources you need without altering the meaning, and present the gist of the sources in your own words to support your writing.

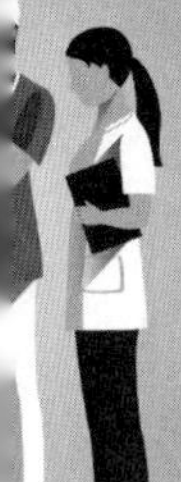

Unit 8 Medical Ethics

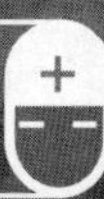

Summarize each of the following paragraphs into one or two sentences after reading the paragraph thoroughly. Underline the key points while reading, then condense and reorganize the key points together after reading.

❶ In 2011, the UN Political Declaration on non-communicable diseases (NCDs) called for population-based policies, multisectoral action, cross-agency working and monitoring and evaluation. The World Health Organization (WHO) has led the way in developing this global response to NCDs. They have put into place a global architecture for addressing NCDs, including recommendations on population-based actions and monitoring frameworks with targets and indicators. Greater coordination is needed between this process and actions being taken to address undernutrition and challenges in the food system at the global, regional and national levels. NCDs have been conspicuously absent from both the health and nutrition-related Millennium Development Goals (MDGs) and other international development agendas. At the national level there has been a wide range of responses, but still insufficient formulation and implementation of integrated policies, cross-sectoral governance, and monitoring and evaluation.

Summary: ____

____

____

____

❷ Traditional medicine, which uses a wide variety of inexpensive, easily accessible, and familiar natural ingredients and techniques, is preferable for many people. Traditional medicines are normally created from local plants, animals, and minerals. Techniques often include socially bonding physical contact between patient and healer like rubbing or massaging, and spiritual experiences which may involve trances, music, and scents. In Africa, for instance, an estimated 80% of people rely on traditional medicine for almost all their health care. Similarly, in many other parts of the world, particularly in Asia and Latin America where modern facilities are available, this approach to medicine is still highly valued because it is effective, inexpensive, and culturally significant.

Summary: ____

____

____

____

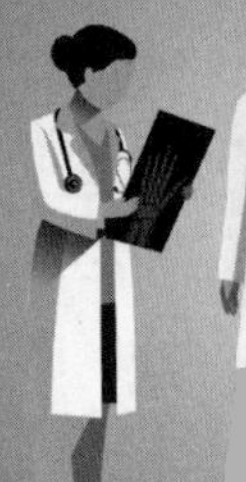

❸ Comprehensive palliative care services integrate the expertise of a team of providers from different disciplines to address the complex needs of seriously ill patients and their families. Members of a palliative care team typically include professionals from medicine, nursing, and social work, with additional support from chaplaincy and professionals in nutrition, rehabilitation, pharmacy, and other professional disciplines, as needed. These programs are now available at more than 80% of large US hospitals (those with more than 300 beds), where most Americans receive their care during complex and advanced illness.

Despite the increasing availability of palliative care services in US hospitals and the body of evidence showing the great distress to patients caused by symptoms of the illness, the burdens on family caregivers, and the overuse of costly, ineffective therapies during advanced chronic illness, the use of palliative care services by physicians for their patients remains low. Physicians tend to perceive palliative care as the alternative to life-prolonging or curative care—what we do when there is nothing more that we can do—rather than as a simultaneously delivered adjunct to disease-focused treatment.

Summary: ____

____

____

____

➢ To find more information about summarizing, you may refer to the following sources.

1. McCombes, S. 2020. How to write a summary guide & examples. Retrieved January 17, 2021, from Scribbr website.
2. Smith, S. 2022. Summarizing. Retrieved February 28, 2022, from EAP Foundation website.